CONTENTS

35 Kg = + 42 Km

FROM OBESITY TO MARATHON RUNNER

FABIANO PUPO BARBOSA BIANCHI

2016

Original Title: Da Obesidade à Maratona

English version by Mari Trevisan

Proofreading by Mari Trevisan

INTRODUCTION

When I decided to write this book, I wanted to share my experience with losing weight and becoming a runner, or more accurately, a marathoner. I wanted to talk about how I left a sedentary lifestyle to become a cheerful runner.

I decided to publish a book because many of my friends, upon hearing my story, insisted that I shared it on a blog or on a social network, since it was such a motivating and realistic experience.

Everyone seemed very interested in my experience, so many questions came and I started giving advice on running. The best part was that many people started running after talking to me.

I opted for a book because it is a simpler way of sharing everything: my story, facts and many situations and occurrences that may prove useful to those who wish to venture into this amazing life of running.

I believe that it is important to emphasise that what I will be describing in this book has no scientific basis, no medical research, and neither nutritionist nor healthcare professional instruction. Everything contained here is just *my* experience, including my hits and misses and my experiments and tests.

Perhaps many of the things I did or practised were terribly wrong, but it all worked out for me. I drew onthorough internet research, my own studies and many obvious conclusions, plus huge result observation.

I did not write this book in order to sell any magical or fast weight loss formula. I am just going to share here what I did and how I did it, nothing more than that. I will describe a period of my life in which I managed to rebuild my self-esteem through cheap, regular exercise. I believe that the results I have obtained have been so satisfying that many have congratulated me and thanked me for being a source of motivation for them.

However, I do not intend to make you follow my steps. That is not my intention. I just wish to share my experience so that it may motivate you and show you that willpower is all it takes to boostyour results.

I beg your pardon for my technical ignorance, since as I mentioned, I did not consult with any healthcare professional and I have no formal training in this field. I'm just a strong-willed person!

Before sharing my experience with you, I believe that it is vital to make a brief description of what I was going through and how my life was like before I started running.

I had turned 40 years old in September 2014 and on the ten days that followed my birthday that year, my life took a turn for the worse. I had moved to Ubatuba – a city in the northern coast of the state of São Paulo –a year and a half before that period and my wife was still living in our apartment in São Paulo. We managed to sell our apartment a week before my birthday, which would enable my wife to move permanently to Ubatuba. Everything was going smoothly. I had started making plans to revamp my house as I was just waiting to receive our down payment. However,as life would have it, my marriage ended nine days after my birthday, for reasons that are indifferent to this story, and since I'm a lucky guy, the buyer of our apartment had his loan refused and thus the sale was cancelled.

The following months were terrible. Divorcing is never easy, my restaurant in Ubatuba was barely scraping by, and with the economic crisis that Brazil was going through, I could not have any goodexpectations. I was starting to worry about my imminent lack of money. Moreover, my loneliness and memories of my marriage also made me feel depressed.

At this point, I no longer had any concern with beauty or aesthetics. I would eat indiscriminately and drunkenness, as well as partying all night, became more and more common. It was usual for me to get home inebriated and so I started gaining weight fast. I used to weigh 98 kg, but it quickly reached 107 kg.

As months went by, the false idea that I was over my divorce settled in and I felt that desperate need to find a new match. My weekend parties became weekday parties as well. As a result, my sleep schedule was ruined, causing me to work while drowsy and thus making mistakes. By then, I knew that something was wrong and that I needed to do something about it soon.

Everything started to change after the 2015 Carnival, when I went out with a childhood friend who had come to Ubatuba to visit his brother. He came to my house and we walked to a nearby club. We had a very pleasant night; we met several friends and ended up going out together. I felt good. I was wearing new clothes. I have always considered myself an attractive man, and it was very usual to see women interested in me. I was handsome that night, or at least I felt that way, since I was very well dressed and felt happy. As the night ended, I had only managed to get drunk. We went back home and I said goodbye to my friend. Something was off, but I couldn't put my finger on it.I had a restless sleep. I do not remember what I dreamed of, but it must not have been good, because I woke up scared.

I could not forget that night when I woke up the next morning. What happened? What was wrong with me? What surprised me the most was that no woman had looked at me during the party. That really bothered me. I always considered myself attractive, and flirting with a woman during a party was something that usually happened. That day there was no such thing, and it bothered me, by the way, that night bothered me for a few weeks after that.

In early March 2015, I went to São Paulo to sign my divorce papers. In that same month, I sold my apartment, so I had less things to worry about. I was still weighing over 107 kg, though, and I needed to focus on running my restaurant, since business was still slow. I bought a few sports shorts and t-shirts in São Paulo, and was thinking about using my old dumbbells again. I did not realise then that that was probably a sign for what was to come.

I went back home determined to start working out. The first day when I was supposed to get up early, I turned off my alarm and went back to sleep. "I'll start tomorrow", I said to myself. The problem was that "tomorrow" became "next week", and so on. My dumbbells still lay on the floor, unused.

One fine day, around the beginning of the second half of March, as I got out of bed, I looked at myself in the mirror. I had just woken up and I looked awful. To make matters worse, I was wearing very old boxers with frayed elastics. "Homer Simpson!" was the first thing that crossed my mind. I did not know whether to laugh or cry... I cried. I was the personification of Jabba The Hut. Fat. Ugly. Old. Helpless. I looked like I was dirty. Who would want me like that? "No one!" I said to myself.

In that moment, I wallowed in self-hate. How could I let my body stay that way? What kind of life was I planning – or rather, how did I want to die?

Suddenly, many explanations popped up in my mind. "That is why you cannot find a girlfriend anymore. You are ugly. That is why you get tired. You are fat." I had not realised it until then, but as I cursed at myself, I needed to sit down and place one leg on top of the other just to tie my shoelaces. "That's why my shoelaces were always placed on the sides of my shoes." It was obvious that all of it needed to change, but how? What should I do?

CHAPTER I – THE REASON AND THE CHOICE

I had decided: I needed to lose weight anyway and I wanted it to happen soon. I still didn't know how to do it, though. I still had not made my decision.

The first thing I did was to look for gyms in Ubatuba and the majority of the answers I got was: "You are too overweight to work out. Let's start by walking on a treadmill." I realised that I would spend months renting the gym's treadmill. I gave up.

I had an epiphany on a cloudy day, when I was walking with Vicky Hound (my Basset Hound) on the shore of Cruzeiro beach. A group of women in their forties was exercising nearby. There was an instructor with them, who gave the women all the exercises that they had to do on the beach, and they complained all the time. All of them were overweight and it was easy to see that they were struggling.

I stood there for a few minutes watching the group struggle with each exercise, when all of sudden a thin, fast-paced silhouette appeared on the shore. It was a man in his thirties, wearing nylon shorts and a tank top from a marathon. He was running on the shore, and as he approached the women, he shouted out to them: "You want to lose weight? You should run!" and he disappeared just as he had appeared, with quick and light footfalls. It was almost like he was floating.

That affected me. I am not sure why, but it did. "I'll start running." That man had given me the solution I needed.

I went home thinking about how I would start exercising. I needed shorts, t-shirts and sneakers. I had bought shorts and t-shirts in São Paulo, and although my sneakers weren't exactly new, they were good enough to start running.

Having decided to start my weight loss journey on the next day, I started making preparations.

I downloaded a playlist on my iPhone, which I intended to use as a walkman. I bought an armband to attach it to my arm while exercising and I also installed an app to monitor my workout. I set my alarm to six in the morning and laid out my workout clothes. I decided not to tell anyone, lest I give up, saying: "I knew it! It was just a flash in the pan!"

Everything was ready, but it begged the question: "ready for what?" I knew that I wasn't fit enough to run. Actually, I was aware of my size and of how much I could be injured if I tried to run with all that weight. I would have to start by walking. How much should I walk? At what speed? Since I had no knowledge of this, I decided to exercise for at least an hour and I had to return home all sweaty. That was my parameter. I chose to walk from my house, which is in Professor Chico Santos Avenue, to the old Caisão[1]of Ubatuba. This route was about 3.7 km (7.4 km round-trip), which I intended to complete in an hour.

That was it, then. I really needed to take care of myself. I knew that, if I didn't do anything, my situation would

---

[1] "Caisão" is a popular name for the Ubatuba docks. It is a historical place and it provides visitors with one of the most beautiful views of the Ubatuba Bay.

only get worse. The depression monster was already lurking around my house and it was quickly becoming a cave.

Although this may seem funny to most people, the fact that you live near the beach does not mean that your life is wonderful. This is a great mistake. Life near the beach is much more difficult than life in the city. Job opportunities and consequently salaries are absurdly lower than in the city and while I do believe that you need less when living in a small city in the country or on the coast, it is very difficult to earnthis "less". Moreover, living in a city on your own, away from family and childhood friends, can make you feel lonely. Loneliness and lack of money usually make people more dedicated to their jobs, and as a result they feel even more exhausted. There comes a time when you start going "from home to work and from work to home." If you are not careful, this is when the depression monster comes into your home. You are already fed up with work and you are stuck at home all day. Eating, sleeping, and sullying the home that you haven't cleaned in weeks. The stage is set for the spectacle of depression.

I found myself very close to this stage when I saw my reflection in that mirror. Not only did I look awful, but my soul was already stained by the depression monster. I no longer cared about my appearance. My hair was long and unkempt. My beard was unruly and unshaven. My clothes were singed and stained. I spent all my days off work sorry about myself, my divorce and complaining that life was bad. I no longer cleaned my house and it was slowly becoming a cave, dark, sullen and musty. I didn't leave home anymore. I didn't go to the beach anymore. I was ashamed of my body. I started hiding under that "poor little thing" façade.

My motivation to start running was the future I envisioned. I wanted to be thin and to have a healthy, beautiful body. I wanted to be cheerful and friendly, happy with myself and with my life. I wanted to have an orderly, clean, organised house, thus chasing the depression monster away.

CHAPTER II – THE BEGINNING – (MY FIRST STEPS)

My alarm rang at six in the morning. It was bright outside. The first thing that crossed my mind was: "I'm not going."

This is one of the biggest problems that we face: laziness! Laziness will always be your enemy. Just like an obsessive thought, laziness is always present. Many times, after running two kilometres, I felt laziness compelling me to return home and to climb into my bed. It is always there, and don't you think that it goes away with me, for that is a lie. Just let yourself relax for a few days and it will come back in full force. That's why it is so difficult to go back to doing an activity. The word that you have to use to fight laziness is *focus*! It is never acceptable to lose a battle due to laziness.

I opened my eyes to see my simple alarm ringing. I didn't think twice. I hit the small black button and turned it off. I jumped out of bed and put on the workout clothes that were laid out on my desk. I felt that soothing morning chill when I got out of bed. I had just a glass of sugar-free lemon mate tea. I put my phone in my armband and attached it to my arm.

I opened the gate and left. I stretched for a bit on the sidewalk, leaning on a garbage bin. I won't lie, I only do three stretches – one for my calf, one for the back of my leg and one for my thigh. To this day, after years of running, I do the same three stretches. However, I do all of them correctly, without haste and stretching the best I can.

I turned on the app that would monitor my workout. I put on my earphones. I chose a song from my playlist and left. I started by walking slowly. The idea of having a route to be completed in a certain amount of time made me quickly set a pace. I knew that I had to get to the end of the route in half an hour, and thus I'd be able to complete it in an hour.

The stunning view of the Ubatuba shore and the music helped distract me and keep me from thinking about the remaining distance. I managed to complete the 7.5 km route in an hour and twelve minutes, which meant an average walking pace of 9'30"/Km. I didn't know if that was a good pace, but I had come back home as planned… sweating! I now had a time-based walk to beat.

That morning workout had made me feel confident. I was in a good mood and feeling motivated. I even looked in the mirror, trying to notice any minuscule change in my body. I didn't want to tell anyone just yet – I decided to keep it secret because many people are quick to discourage others. In fact, I was told the following many times: "You want to wake up early to work out? You'll stop soon..." or "I bet you won't work out when it rains," and many other sentences that cannot affect your FOCUS in any way. I'll confess: I enjoy running in bad weather – cloudy, drizzly, cold days, those are my favourite days to run.

I woke up on the next day before my alarm rang. I quickly put my clothes on and left. This time I used the app more carefully, trying to improve my walking time, and so I kept a slightly higher average pace. I managed to improve it by a minute.

One of the things I mostly enjoyed doing when I started walking was to choose a destination, which I called "waypoint", as I read on sailing books. That's what they called their intermediate stops. Choosing a waypoint is merely psychological, but extremely useful, since you not only needn't look at a watch nor GPS all the time, but also you cannot cheat on your workout. When I get to my waypoint (Ubatuba's Caisão), I always step on its concrete floor as a way of confirming that I actually *stepped* on my waypoint. I needn't say how cool it is when you choose a waypoint and start seeing it in the distance after a while. That gives me renewed strength to complete my personal challenge.

Nowadays, I use Google Maps to choose my waypoints and set my routes. Firstly, I choose the distance I want to walk and then I calculate the time that it would take. At this point, one should have several things in mind, such as: "Is it round trip? If it is just one way, how will I come back? Is there public transportation on the way back? Should I take some money? Will I need to pack water or something to eat? Are there any nearby shops? Should I take my mobile phone?" Finally, to avoid any complications, one should think of the smallest details. Many complicated, common things may happen when you are far away from home, such as an injury. Imagine if you are more than twenty kilometres away from home, with no mobile phone, no money, at dawn, and then you sprain your ankle and can barely walk. If my workouts are far from the city, for instance, in an isolated place, I always take money, water and my phone with me. I always let someone know my route and when I'm leaving. It is better to be safe than sorry.

It is vital to choose a route and a waypoint when you are starting out. If you are able to find a waypoint during your workout time, without needing to repeat the route, that is great. I am not sure why, but walking or running without a destination is a bit dull and exhausting, since the workout only comes down to time, then, and that might make you keep checking your watch every five minutes.I recall that my first few walks were something like "I'm going to walk to the Caisão today. Tomorrow, I'm going to walk to the end of the Perequê-Açu beach." There was always a destination and that always made me finish a workout, no matter how tired I was. When we see our destination, a force comes from deep within our core and pushes us for a few more kilometres.

If you are planning to start running one day, choose a route and a waypoint. Use an app, a GPS, a map, a website, anything, but it is most important not to be surprised by the distance, nor by the places you will pass by.

I was excited about my willingness to walk and thus started a routine. I would wake up around five in the morning, got ready and started working out. I returned home and took Vicky for a walk. Afterwards, I would shower and go to work. I'd feel tired when I returned home around 6 PM. Mission accomplished. I would shower again, grab something to eat and go to bed at 9 PM. The quality of my sleep improved and so did my stamina. I now cared again about my looks and about tidying up my house.

It was amazing how exercising had changed my life so much.

CHAPTER III – STARTING TO LOSE WEIGHT

I now had a routine, and most importantly, I was focused. Waking up at dawn became a habit to me. I was used to working out when it was still dark, and thus I would watch the sunrise. That was a gift and a privilege of living on the coast. The sunrise was a daily, beautiful spectacle. I wanted to watch the sunrise every day, so that made me feel more motivated to get up and get ready to leave. It is magnificent to run on the Itaguá shore while seeing the sun rising in the horizon, reflecting its rays on the sea. Birds flying, fishing boats floating, the vegetation along the shoreline, the sound of the waves. Everything makes up one of the most beautiful landscapes I have ever seen, and even though I see it every day, I never get bored – I'm just thankful for this privilege.

It had been almost a month since I'd started walking, and I could not hide it anymore, for it started to show. One day I was at work when a customer said: "You look thinner. Are you on a diet? You look healthier." I told him I had started walking, so that could be it. My team heard him and also said that I looked thinner.

I was curious. "Did I really lose weight?" I could not stop thinking about it. After leaving work, I visited a drugstore and weighed myself. 100 kilos! I got off the scale and weighed myself again and again, I couldn't believe it! I had lost 5 kg. I felt happy, excited, overjoyed. It was working.

I visited two more drugstores on my way home, but I was let down. In one of them, I weighed 102 kg and 99 kg in the other one. I realised that there is a difference between scales and that my clothes also interfered in my weight. I'd have to weigh myself without any clothes on and always at the same time. I left the last drugstore with a small scale in my hands. From that day forward, I started weighing myself without any clothes on, after working out, before showering. Later, I also started weighing myself before working out, so that I'd know much weight I'd lose per work out, by dehydration.

It is common to lose a lot of weight just after starting working out – usually around five kilos. You may have heard someone say: "It's easy to lose five kilos!" It is really easy to lose those first five kilograms. I believe that is an excessive weight that our bodies try to eliminate as fast as possible.I needn't say how motivated I was when I lost those first few kilos.

Even though was my life was pretty much the same, I felt thin again and that everyone would notice it, and then they would compliment me for it. I felt attractive, energetic, and younger. It was nothing but an illusion, though. It wasn't possible to notice any changes in my body yet, especially for those who saw me almost daily. More importantly, it was a personal achievement. When someone noticed that something was different and asked me about it, I would simply beam with pride and say: "Yes! I lost five kilos."

Fast weight loss can be very encouraging, but do not fool yourself. It will take much longer to lose more weight, and that *is* indeed discouraging! That's why I insist that you must remain *focused*. We must not give up our goals. Even though it is vital to keep track of your weight, most people say: "don't weigh yourself every day!" I personally disagree, since I do weigh myself every day, but you should weigh yourself every week or every ten days, since it is a lot more reassuring to see that you lost more than you had anticipated.

We can lose weight in a very busy day, and so can we gain weight on a weekend out with friends, beer, food and lack of exercise. Again, it is discouraging to see that you gained two kilos after a night out. The truth is that our bodies tend to keep a "water weight" of four kilos, which varies depending on our daily activities. Therefore, you can gain two kilos after a night out, and it is also possible to lose some weight after working out all day. This is why weighing yourself daily is not recommended.

I had lost five kilos, and I knew it wasn't part of this "water weight" – I knew it because I'd weigh myself almost daily, even more so after people noticed that I was thinner. I would weigh 102 kilos on a day, then 103 kilos the next day. A few days later, my weight would vary between 101 and 103 kilos, then all of a sudden 100 kilos. A few days passed, then my weight varied again until it reached 99 kg. This is how I realised that I was losing weight.

My walking time also improved with weight loss. I had been able to reduce almost ten minutes of my course record. I had become faster and lighter, and with that I could walk faster. As I mentioned before, I stopped losing weight after losing those first five kilos, or so I'd thought. Sometimes it seemed like I wasn't losing weight and that was frustrating. "Will I only be able to lose five kilos after a month of exercising?" I decided it was time to focus on my diet as well, which hadn't changed at all until then.

I had terrible eating habits. I would eat junk food and healthy food, so despite eating salads, meats, grains and drinking natural juices, I would also eat pizzas, hamburgers, soft drinks, ice-cream, industrialised snacks and all kinds of food that someone wishing to have a heart attack should eat. I realised that I could lose a few more kilos if I managed to improve my awful eating habits. However, I didn't want to go on a diet – I just wanted to eat less, so instead of eating three loaves of bread for breakfast, I'd eat just one. Instead of eating four slices of pizza, I'd eat just two. While I reduced all my food portions by half, I did not cut out any foods to lose weight.

This was indeed a great strategy, since I continued to gradually lose weight without missing any goodies nor any kinds of food. I wanted to reduced my food portions based on the thought "eat less and spend more." The idea, then, was to keep spending my concentrated source of energy (fat) without replenishing it, and it worked. In doing so, I managed to lose almost five more kilos, so I weighed 96 kgnow.

Finally, the difference was clear, since I was almost ten kilos thinner – people commented on it, my clothes were baggier, and even my snoring was reduced. I used to snore a lot, and losing weight made me stop snoring. Everything seemed to be going smoothly, so much so that I got to date a girl at a party, and so my self-esteem also improved. However, all good things come to an end: it became difficult to lose weight after I'd reached 95 kg.

I didn't know why I wouldn't lose weight anymore. I kept walking faster and faster and kept controlling my eating habits, but those 95 kg would still show up on my scale. I still had a long way to go to reach my goal of 80kg, so I could not afford to stop losing weight.

CHAPTER IV – FROM WALKING TO RUNNING

I did not manage to lose any more weight, even though I kept following my routine. Walking, taking Vicky for a walk, work, eating less, no parties, no alcohol. It was frustrating, mostly because I knew what options I had. I could try a stricter diet or I could improve my walking workouts. I won't lie, neither option seemed exciting, but I knew what I needed to do. I didn't want to change my eating habits again, since I loved eating – I didn't want to give up the foods that made me happy. In my mind, improving my workouts meant enrolling in a gym, but I was not willing to spend money nor to feel embarrassed when exercising next to six-pack men and women. I definitely did not want to compare myself to such people. I needed to change my habits and start losing weight again, preferably without spending money.

Everything started to change without me having to find out how. On a fine day in April, about a month and a half after I'd started working out, I was following my routine as usual. I woke up early and had my phone, my hat and my sunglasses on me. I left home, stretched and started walking, just like every other day. I recall that I had a pace of 7:40 minutes per kilometre, which means that I could walk pretty fast. If I walked a bit faster, perhaps I could start running. The more I walked, the more my legs wanted to accelerate. I was starting to think about running. How would I do that? How long would I try to run?

On that first day, I used signs, poles and bends on the road as waypoints, for example: "I will try to run to that pole, or to that sign." I managed to run short distances. I actually had no idea what the distance was to that pole or that sign, but I ran there nonetheless. I was sure that I'd have a heart attack or a stroke, since my lungs seemed to pop out of my mouth. I did think I'd black out, but I did not – I survived!

When I got back home, I wanted to check how much I'd run, so I had set two points of reference which I could easily locate on Google Maps. From McDonald's to Praça da Baleia and after a month and a half of daily walking, I had run merely 350 METRES! What a pitiful result.

I really wanted to start running, but I was afraid it was too early to risk it. I have always been too scared of injuring myself, I was already 40 years old and in this age one cannot recover as fast as when one is young. There's something very interesting that my brother says about getting old: "When you are young and crash your motorbike, you get up, beat off the dust, climb back on it and leave. When you're older, you wake up with a lot of back pain after sleeping in your own bed." This is accurate – when you reach a certain age (in my opinion, after thirty-five years old), you have to be much more careful. A tendon or knee injury or even fractures might not completely heal, so I didn't want to risk injuring myself by running while overweight.

The fact that I'd managed to run 350 metres also motivated me to risk a few bursts. I just had to plan a way of starting slowly, without being hard on myself and with enough time to recover. I was using the Nike app to monitor my walks, and it communicates through an automatic voice every time I completed a kilometre. Each time I walk a kilometre, I'd run 300 metres. I just needed to pay attention to the updates on my mobile phone, and so I placed it on my forearm. As soon as I walked a kilometre, I'd start running.

I decided to try it on the next day. I woke up very early, got dressed, left, stretched and started walking. I was overcome by fear and anxiety, though. I feared the unknown and how my body would respond to this new activity, and my anxiety made the app useless, since I checked my phone every fifty metres. "One kilometre. Time. 7 minutes, 40 seconds. Speed 7.38. Average Speed 7.38." That was the notification. "It's now or never", I thought. "Alright then, let's start running."

I took a deep breath, tilted my torso a bit and raised my right knee. A long stride of my right leg and an impulsion with my left calf started my run. That first step changed everything, and I would only realise that many months later. In that small push, in that small step, I had started the biggest and best change that my body would go through in many years. In that moment, I was Neil Armstrong and that was my "giant leap for mankind". I was running. Stride after stride, breath after breath and I kept going, metre by metre. I would be running for at least 300 metres.

When one starts running, everything seems a bit fuzzy. It is common to be under the impression that one is running crookedly, or unbalanced. One worries about their breath, or more accurately, about breathing correctly, as they teach us in P.E. classes in school. You have to inhale through your nose and exhale through your mouth. Inhale through the nose and exhale through the mouth. Inhale through the nose and exhale through the mouth. Inhale through the nose and exhale through the mouth. Phew! I still felt that unbearable pain on the side of the abdomen, which is attributed to breathing in the wrong way during running.

I later found that all that talk about breathing correctly, in one way or another, is a lie. We are all different, so there isn't one way for all of us to breathe. In fact, I barely breathe through my right nostril and I am not sure whether it is due to a deviated septum or not, I just know that I can't breathe very well through it.Therefore, this technique of inhaling through the nose and exhaling through the mouth did not work out well for me. However, I found that the human body always find a way to adapt. I was very worried about my breathing at first and thus had that side pain bother me a lot. I started thinking: "Relax. It'll sort itself out". I let my body solve the problem and find a way to breathe. It worked. Nowadays, I inhale and exhale through my mouth in a paced way. I don't feel that pain anymore nor do I get tired quickly. My body has found a way to adapt.

I got tired before completing two hundred metres. I was so tired that I felt like a heart attack was imminent. When I completed two hundred and fifty metres, I did take my eyes off my phone. Each and every metre was being agonizingly monitored.

Three hundred metres! I did it! I think I didn't shout that out loud, but I would not doubt it if someone said that I did, so great was my exhaustion and my excitement to complete that short – but at the time, infinite – distance. I had managed to complete that first run. It was my first run because I'd start running again seven hundred metres from there and meanwhile, I had to rest.I believe it is unnecessary to say that I felt scared again when I was close to walking two kilometres.

That was how running went like on that day; I walked seven kilometres between three hundred metres bursts and seven hundred metres walks. In total, I ran two kilometres and a hundred metres, and that result made me very happy.

By analysing app data, I realised that even though I ran two kilometres, my time had not changed much. I noticed that my walks were slower as a result of the exhaustion caused by running. I did not worry about that, though, for I knew that I would improve my performance and that in due time, I'd be able to walk as fast as before and that my total elapsed time would be much shorter.

My walking and running plan continued and I gradually improved it. After a few days of running three hundred metres, I started running five hundred metres, and consequently my elapsed time was shortened as I lost more weight.

I could now run five hundred metres for each kilometre that I walked and that was an incredible achievement. My exhaustion had increased and my sleep greatly improved, and so did my stamina. I felt like a new person, I was physically changing and my good mood was noticeable, so much so that people started asking: "What happened? You seem very happy!".

I now weighed 92 kilos due to my new workout routine, but then I stopped losing weight again. I was already very happy that I had lost more than ten kilos rather quickly and without any professional help. After a few weeks, my five hundred metres runs were conducted without any pain nor complaints; on the contrary, I'd excitedly wait for the app to notify me so that I could start running. Thus, I decided it was time to be a bit bolder. "I'm able to run around 3.5 km now, so what if I tried to run that distance without stopping?" That doubt had been tormenting me for a while and I was willing to try it.

It was early May when I decided to risk a longer run. I decided to run back home from the Ubatuba Yatch Club, roughly two kilometres long.I ran those two kilometres with no difficulty. I had succeeded! I felt incredible, like a hero, like Superman. I had run two kilometres and I was feeling well, with no pain nor exhaustion. It was time to try harder. I decided to run from the Caisão to my house on the next day, a route of 3.5 km and a few metres. I reached my goal again. It was time to try to complete my walkingroute by running.

I was planning to run the 7.5 km and a half distance between my house and the Caisão (round trip). I would run with a lot of care, so that I wouldn't be injured.

I put my plan into practice on the next day, and I managed to complete the route a lot easily than I had anticipated. What I feared – failure, hurting myself, making a fool of myself – was only in my head rather than being real. Once, a friend of mine, who would later become my running partner, Zildo Lopes, told me something that helped me overcome that willingness to give up running. He said: "Fabi, it is when you cannot take it anymore, when your body is begging you to stop, that you must press on. Tell yourself that you are going to run just a few more metres. Then you keep going. Your body will get used to it soon and you will be able to continue." Zildo was right. I went through that giving up period, which usually occurs in the first three kilometres, and then I kept going. I told myself that I could not stop and I was sure that my body would get used to the exercise. And so it was – I managed to complete my route in less than an hour. I was over the moon. *I managed to run seven kilometres*! I had never imagined I would be able to run 7 km non-stop.

From that day forward, seven kilometres and a half was the shortest distance that I would run. From home to the Caisão and back.

CHAPTER V – LOSING WEIGHT FASTER

As my daily walks progressed to 7 kilometre runs, losing weight was inevitable. I now weighed 86 kilos. My clothes were a lot baggier and some of my trousers and t-shirts did not fit anymore. Although I used to hate shopping for clothes, it had become a reason to celebrate my weight loss.

I loved being praised and I was proud to talk about my achievements and about how much weight I'd lost. That's important – when you achieve something, find a way for people to know it: mention your achievements during a conversation, or do it when someone notices your progress. It is extremely encouraging to be complimented or to see people surprised by the distance you ran, since not onlyyou'll feel rewarded for your hard work, but you will also be much more focused and determined to reach your goals. Never stop talking about your achievements, for although there will be negative comments, you will also feel support and praise, which you must always remember.

I now weighed 86 kg and I had stopped losing weight again. That worried me, because I did not know to lose weight anymore – I ran, I ate less food. What else should I do? I knew that I could try changing my eating habits, such as cutting greasy food and flour out of my diet. I could also try running more, since perhaps running less than fifty minutes a day was not enough. However, I wasn't willing to try any of those options. I insisted on my normal routine for another week, but the numbers on my scale wouldn't change. There was no apparent solution.

One day, after running in a stormy morning and seeing that my weight did not change, I decided to try both options, since there was no other way. I would create a longer route and I would start a very-low-calorie diet (VLCD). I managed to create a meal plan after doing some research. It contained liquids, salads, fruit and meats. I was sure that following that diet, along with intense workout, would make me lose more weight.

As a result of my new diet, I started feeling lazier, sleepier and much more tired after exercising, not to mention that I would get as hungry as a bear. My average pace had also increased. In other words, my performance had worsened a lot and I would not have it. As much as I was disappointed about my new performance, it was clear that the weight loss I so desperately wanted was making me weak. In order to find a solution, I visited a dietary supplements store and told them about my problem.

A very helpful retailer introduced me to a supplement that I still use to this day – a caffeine-based thermogenic supplement that renewed my willingness to run, especially during my workout sessions. I would take a pill half an hour before running and another one hour after exercising. It gave me extra energy during my runs and it also kept me going throughout the day. According to the retailer, the supplement burned fats on the adipose tissue in the gluteus and in the abdomen, and being caffeine-based meant that it would make me more active during the day. Incredibly enough, the pills worked just like she said they would.

My abdomen got ripped and I felt more energized. Furthermore, I combined that thermogenic supplement with a vitamin supplement, since I was afraid I wasn't consuming enough vitamins due to the changes in my diet. I believe it is vital to contact a health professional before taking supplements and vitamins, though I didn't do it myself. My strategy was indeed successful. I was able to run just like before and I never got the flu again. I have been running for years now, and I have not gotten sick ever since. I am also able to run in any weather, be it rainy, sunny, stormy, cold, etc. I am positive that my immunity is a result of that vitamin complex – I still take a pill every single day, even on days when I do not work out.

I had one thing in mind – I knew that I could do without rice, beans, fried food, breads and potatoes, but not without meat. On the contrary, I doubled my meat consumption. Now that I ingested less than a thousand calories a day, my weight indeed dropped, to the point that I had bits of loose skin on the sides of my body. At this point, I'd lose weight almost daily. I decided, then, to put the second part of my strategy into practice: I would run farther.

I could now complete my original route in less than forty-five minutes and had to keep running for at least an hour. As I intended to increase the amount of exercise, I decided to simply double my route. I would go to the Caisão twice, which would give better time and greater distance to cover.

On the next day, I was very excited about that new challenge. For the first time, I'd run more than ten kilometres. Along with my excitement, however, I also feared the unknown. "Can I do it?" that question burned in my mind. I wanted to test myself. As usual, I got up when my alarm went off, dressed, left, stretched and started running – this time, a much longer route.

I was on the verge of completing my course within my course record, but this time I was not feeling tired. I decided to take a turn and return to the Caisão when I reached the newsstand near Praça da Baleia. On that moment, that newsstand became one of my waypoints, since I'd always return there. I stepped on the Caisão and made my way back home.

I got home having completed the course in an hour and a half, which was a good time. I was as tired as when I completed that course for the first time, but I was also very happy. I was even more surprised when I weighed myself and found that I'd lost yet another kilogram in hat run. I knew that the amount of liquid that I'd lost would be replaced, but I had surely lost some fat as well.

That longer run made me feel tired all day. I was feeling well, but I felt sleepy. When I got home from work, I took a shower and ended up taking a nap on my couch, while watching TV. I decided to rest my body for a day, as I had pushed it too hard. I did not run on the next day.

I went back to running after that day-long rest. I ran those thirteen kilometres again and this time, it was not so difficult. After repeating that course a few times, my body had seemingly got used to it. On a lazy day, I ended up running only half the course, but I thought it insufficient after completing those seven kilometres in less than forty minutes. From that day forward, I would only leave home to run for more than an hour. My goal had always been time, not distance. The minimum amount of daily exercise for me should be an hour, and I wasn't interested in leaving home if I was only able to exercise for less than an hour.

Now that I ran thirteen kilometre and followed my VLC diet, I started losing a lot of weight and thus reached 80 kilos in the blink of an eye. But my weight loss did not stop there. I kept losing weight until I reached 75 kg. My time improved a lot, my pace was around 5:10, which was an excellent time for someone who had started running only a few months prior. I also started trying to run 15 kilometres by leaving home on the Itaguá district and running all the way to the end of Perequê-Açu beach (I ran to the Indaiá River, where the road ends), to the Caisão then back home. That route was around 15 kilometres.

As a result of the huge increase in physical activity and calorie reduction, my fitness, sleep, metabolism and even digestive system improved. My hair had never been so straight and even um skin improved. Please note that I mentioned "calorie reduction", not diet reduction. Although 800 calories per day might not seem enough, it is possible to have feasts if one eats low-calorie food. My food portions were much bigger than in the past. I started using salad bowls as plates, since I'd eat big portions of salad during my meals. I would be lying if I told you that I was still hungry when I left the table. On the contrary, many times I could not even finish eating. All I had to do was to change what I ate. Instead of rice and beans, I ate lettuce, rockets, tomatoes, cucumbers, etc. Instead of regular soft drinks, I drank sugar-free soft drinks, and as for dessert… well, those were never part of my diet.

After a month of running around thirteen kilometres and a half five days a week (67.5 Km a week or 303.75 Km a month), I had a completely different body from when I'd started. I did not have much belly fat anymore and my abdomen was getting ripped. "Who would have thought that I would have a six pack at this age?", it was funny to me. I was very happy with myself, even though I'd had to spend a fortune on clothes, since nothing I owned fit me anymore, not even bathing suits nor underwear. There wasn't a day when I wasn't praised, answered questions about exercising or gave tips on how to lose weight. Many people seemed interested in my achievements and in how I had managed to lose so much weight.

The change my body went through (or perhaps I *had* been very fat indeed) was so great that people that had not seen me in a couple of months did not recognise me. There were funny situations such as when a client asked my brother if I'd left the store. My brother replied: "No. He is right behind the counter." The client was puzzled and said out loud: "You are lying. Is that your brother?".

Once, I decided to shave my head and became completely bald. People asked me if I was sick or perhaps undergoing chemotherapy, since I was very thin and bald. I told them no and I explained to them that I had shaved my head due to the current hot weather. In fact, they asked me that so many times that I never shaved my head again. To be honest, even my sister though it was strange, since she had not seen me in six months – I had lost thirty kilos since the last time we had seen each other. My face and my arms were now slim and I lost that damned excessive skin that only obese people have in the neck area. I changed for the better.

I was so used to running thirteen kilometres that I decided to enter a 10 km race.

CHAPTER VI – MY FIRST 10 KM RACE

I was looking forward to begin participating in races, and I chose start to start by one of Ubatuba's most traditional races, which is called "Soldado Paulino". It is organised by the city's police department as a homage to a former police officer.

This was a 10 km race and even though I was constantly running farther than that, it was impossible not to feel nervous, or anxious about it. Therefore, I decided to get a partner for that race. I talked to my friend Zildo Lopes, who promptly accepted my invitation. I suggested that we ran that course before the date of the race so that I could clear up a few questions that I had, such as: "Are there any steep paths? Can I do it? What about pace?". I invited Zildo because I knew that he'd been running for a while and that he could probably run as fast as I could.

Participating in an official race is very interesting, even more so when you are a beginner. The fact that it is an event, on a certain date and with a certain distance to be covered – which you cannot choose – means that something that you are used to doing becomes a real challenge. As strange as it may seem, one might feel incapable or powerless, the distance to be covered might seem enormous when it is actually shorter than your daily workout; however, our fears and insecurities can create such demons. All these fears actually make the race more exciting. Running for the sake of it is wonderful in its own way, and meeting a passionate group of runners is even more wonderful. Things such as the feeling of being in a race, the weeks prior, specific workouts, the focus, the support from family and friends and finally the end of the race are what makes the thrill of the run even greater.

Entering a race does indeed change one's workout routine entirely. One becomes more compromised to the sport, as one stops skipping workouts. Furthermore, eating habits become stricter and those eight hours of sleep become mandatory. Partying, while once rare becomes non-existent. All of this is very curious, for we start demanding behaviour that should be regular, just because of an event. After I took part on my first race, I never stopped signing up for races, since I got to enjoy counting the days to a race. I would say that I got addicted to running in different places and of having my completion crowned by a medal. Afterwards, comments, compliments, Facebook posts, pictures and congratulations are part of it, too. All of it makes running like a gala party for runners.

I signed up on a website, paid the fee and received the payment confirmation a few days later – along with an application number, my bib number. I was also informed of the date I had to pick up my participation kit. This is the standard procedure for most races. Firstly, you send your registration form through a website, where you must sign up – since many races tend to be organised by the same company, it is easier when you already have an account on their website. Secondly, you must pay the registration fee, which is usually done by bank statement (boletobancário in Brazil) or by credit card. Then you receive an email, which is your confirmation. In this email, there will be important information about your bib number and about the date when you are supposed to get your participation kit, which usually contains the race's official t-shirt, a chip that must be attached to your shoestring (nowadays you can also attach it to your bib number), your bib number with four pins and many sponsor gifts. You can usually pickup your kit two days before the race, and you cannot pick it up on the day of the race.

I did not have any running strategy, also because it would be my first race – I just wanted to complete it without any pain nor exhaustion. That was my goal for the "Soldado Paulino" race.

I changed nothing about my workout. I kept running those 13.5 kilometres almost daily, on that same route from home to the old Caisão. That distance was more than enough for this race, and I was able to lose sufficient calories so that I needn't worry about eating. I would lose around one thousand calories with my workout, and I did not lose much more calories than that on a day. I actually started losing so much weight that I had to pay attention not to go down the 75 kilos mark.

My eating habits were now partially back to normal – I went to back to eating everything (rice, beans, meats, vegetables, fried food and even desserts), under the condition of eating small portions and eating slowly. A friend from work told me to do that and it worked perfectly. When we sit down to eat, it is normal to be famished and anxious about feeling satiated. We practically devour our meal, barely tasting it and we only stop when we so full that we cannot eat a single pea. *That is totally wrong!* That won't necessarily be bad for your health, but it will make you gain a lot of weight. By doing that you are eating much more than you need, and what is left is excessive fat. According to my friend Glaucia Maria da

Silva, this is what you should do: during your meals, get used to putting your fork next to your plate. Every time you put food on your mouth, put the fork next to your plate as you chew and swallow your food. Think about chewing, do not rush it.

Do it throughout your meal and I am sure that you won't be able to clear your plate. The fact is that the information of satiation takes a while to reach the brain, and while it doesn't reach it, we keep eating. When it finally reaches the brain, we have already eaten more food than was necessary. This idea of putting your fork down is nothing but eating slowly, thus giving more time for satiation to reach our brains before we stuff ourselves with food.

I wanted to look stylish on my first race, so I bought brand new running shoes. I was so excited about it that I insisted on telling everyone about the race, and so family and friends were rooting for me. Many people ran into me on the street and asked me about my training, about the date of the race and whether I was preparing. Some people even promised to watch the race (and they did).

This period when I was preparing for my first race was indeed a very happy period of my life. I had managed to lose all the excessive weight – I still had a long way to go before being totally satisfied with my body, but I was pretty content already. Everybody said that I looked good, that I looked five years younger and I looked more handsome. I would receive compliments and encouragement every day. Many people were curious about the methods I'd used to lose weight. There were those who listened attentively, and I was sure that part of my experience would be of use to them, as there were those who criticised me, called me crazy and said that I was lucky not to be sick and that I was playing with my health. It didn't matter. All I knew was that all was good. I'd run almost daily. I'd walk with Vicky. I always went to work in a good mood and that good energy was infectious. My business had improved, so much so that I had new customers every day. My life had entered a safe routine, and only then did I realise how important it was to be disciplined and to create routines.

The race course training day had come. As I previously mentioned, Zildo accepted to train with me, so that we could be prepared for what awaited us. Actually, I wanted to know if I could handle that race, otherwise I would make a fool of myself. as far as I'm concerned, breaking is the biggest shame and the biggest fear of any runner – it means that you were forced to lower your pace or to even stop running due to extreme fatigue. It is normal for a runner to break due to an unexpected injury, but it is indeed shameful when that happens because of exhaustion or overconfidence. That's lack of preparation, disorganisation. I did not want to go through that on my first race. I would never forgive myself if I finished the race walking or worse, if I never got to finish it. In order to improve my self-confidence and also to get used to the course, I invited Zildo for a ten kilometre run.

He arrived at my house at seven in the morning, like we had agreed. He left his car in my street and we walked to the starting point, which was in front of the Military Police battalion – it was near my house. While we made our way there, we exchanged information regarding our best times and we talked about our expectations for the race. We stretched for a bit after arriving there. On our marks, stopwatches set, and we left.

We left from the battalion's entrance gate and turned right on Mar Mediterrâneo Street. We continued through the Vivamar Park neighbourhood to Rio Grande do SulAvenue, downtown direction. We turned on Professor ThomazGalhardo Street, beach direction. We got to the Iperoig Avenue (which is on the shore of Ubatuba Bay). We continued on the direction of the Caisão through the boardwalk. We passed by the ice factory (Gelo Porto), where we turned around and returned. We ran again through the shore avenue to Carlos Drummond de

AndradeAvenue, then we turned right and entered Vivamar Park again. Then, we turned right on the second street and we finally stopped at the gate of the police battalion.

We finished the course in an hour, I was a bit faster and Zildo was a few minutes behind me. The best part was that we managed to finish the course without any excessive fatigue, nor pain neither any complaints. We were definitely ready for the race.

I was happy with the test and confident and I kept training, but now I'd reduced it in the sense that I had stopped trying to improve my time, since I was afraid of injuring myself before the race. It was not necessary to try harder, since the test had convinced me that I would be able to finish the race easily and that any mistake could exclude me from something I had been preparing for with so much effort. And with that, my pace diminished a lot. I kept training almost every day, but now I ran 5:40 per kilometre.

As is the case of any race, this one took place on a Sunday morning (although I only realised later that *all* races take place on Sundays, preferably on mornings). The start is almost always at seven in the morning, for many reasons – first of all, everyone has Sundays off. It is possible to close off streets without compromising traffic, since no one will be late to work. The weather is pleasant in the mornings, since it would be awful to run at midday, with the sun at its peak and too much heat. Interestingly, I only realised those things after my third run. I even thought once: "Whew, Sunday again. Great, I will be able to run."

I walked to the battalion, where the start and end of the race would take place, as it is only a few blocks from home. I noticed something very interesting that would repeat itself in all the races of which I have participated: along the course, other athletes will show up, and they are all going to the same destination as you. The closer I got to the battalion, the more athletes showed up. By the time I was a few metres from the battalion, there were so many runners that we seemed like a bloc on a street parade. That is when one realises how a single event can attract so many people.

The weather was pleasant the event was very well organised. Every race has a common area for runners, which many tend to call "arena." In this place, there's a stage with the podium, various stalls selling sports supplies, event stalls, medical centre, lockers, toilets, sports clubs stalls, etc. This area was very well organised and there were many staff members. The race also contained well-distributed hydration stops along the course. Nowadays, after having completed many races, I can proudly say that Ubatuba has a very well organised 10 km race, which is very pleasant to run.

There is a stretching session just before the race, which is conducted by an instructor from one of the city's gyms. A few minutes before the race, speakers announce how many minutes are left and ask runners to go to the starting line. I must admit that we all feel nervous when we are awaiting the start. Our eyes are fixed on the countdown shown on the big digital watch hanging from the start gate.

5, 4, 3, 2, 1! The starting pistol is fired, the first line of runners, usually composed of elite police officers, dash in front of us, as if they were running the one-hundred metre dash.

The beginning of the race is a very dangerous moment, so much so that a careless runner may compromise his whole race. It's very easy to quicken one's pace – be it for the thrill of the race, or for the fact that one is being left behind – thus not doing as planned and perhaps wasting energy that will be needed on the end of the race. In order to *finish* a race, one must stick to his plan. When I said finish, I really meant it – not lowering your pace, nor walking... I said that without planning, you won't even make it to the finish line. Planning is what will stop you from accelerating unnecessarily. Any race demands planning, even if it's just choosing a pace and keeping it throughout the course. No one can complete a five-kilometre race without having at least mentally prepared themselves. Therefore, a ten kilometre race demands minimal physical and psychological preparation. A fifteen kilometre race or a half-marathon demand good physical and psychological preparation. A marathon *demands* excellent physical preparation, and *especially* psychological preparation.

I tend to say that after twenty kilometres running, our biggest struggle is against our minds, which insist on reminding us that we are tired and that we are not going to make it. I believe that someone who can prepare for a half-marathon, or for a fifteen-kilometre race can also prepare for a marathon. Someone who can run a half-marathon can also run a marathon. The problem lies in psychological preparation. A long race, which is more than thirty kilometres long, is awful torture to those who do not have strong psychological preparation. In my opinion, a person who is able to run twenty kilometres will also be able to run the forty-two kilometres of a marathon, at least physically speaking. The real challenge of a marathon isn't physical... it is psychological. Your mind makes you give up. Your mind and your thoughts defeat you, so that's why it must be trained to deviate from the abdication thoughts that show up along the race.

The first kilometre of the race took place inside Vivamar Park, through its wooded streets and holey asphalt. We ran through one of the main streets of that district, Mar Mediterrâneo Street, which is a long, flat street. On this first kilometre the rule of thumb was to keep my excitement under control and to try and focus on my pace. I had to stick to my running plan. I didn't want to force myself now, I would only try accelerating when I reached the shore. So great was my fear of not completing the race that I almost ran slowly during the first kilometre. Even children were ahead of me, but I kept focused on my pace.

On this first kilometre we entered Rio Grande do SulAvenue until we turned right into Professor ThomazGalhardo Street, and we kept going until we reached the shore. It was at this point that the unprepared, the ones who opted for a fast pace, the older runners and the children stayed behind. This is why it is vital to be careful and not to get overexcited about those who are running for fun and have no willingness to finish the race, for those will fool you into increasing your pace and thus not finishing the race. Of the people that stayed behind, many of them were those who demonstrated the greatest vigour in their first strides.

When I reached the avenue of the shore, my pace was constant and my body had already synchronised my breathing. I was running comfortably. I decided to risk increasing my pace as we crossed the Tavares River and reached Leovigildo Dias Vieira Avenue, also known as Itaguá Avenue. We pressed on to the ice factory that is on the way of the Caisão. I knew that part of the course very well, since it was my daily training ground. I ran faster, for I was feeling confident. We ran four kilometres by the Itaguá shore, to the ice factory and returning to Carlos Drummond de Andrade Avenue, which gives access to Vivamar Park and to the Military Police Battalion. At this point I felt quite tired, but extremely happy, since I was on the verge of completing the race, I did not feel any pain and nothing else would stop me from completing it.

I crossed the finish line in fifty six minutes, a little longer than I was used to running on my workouts. This is pretty common on a race, since there is the messy start and it takes a while to get into your pace and to get enough space to take your strides. Not to mention the fact that you are running under pressure. There are actually many factors behind having a worse time than in one's workouts: the crowd at the start, the other runners that hinder your progress by almost bumping into you or messing up your running pace, the ones that start running and suddenly start walking on the middle of the road and even badly positioned photographers. Everything I mentioned hinders your progress and compromises your final performance.

As this was my first race, I did not care about my best time nor did I care aboutmy final position. What mattered was the fact that I finished the race smoothly, with no pain nor exhaustion. Part of me was laughing cheerfully and wanted to tell everyone that I had managed to finish my first ten kilometre race. I also wanted to let them know that I had lost weight and gained enough resistance to run for ten kilometres non-stop after a few months of training. This was an amazing achievement and I was so euphoric that I only removed the medal when I was about to take a shower.

Zildo Lopes managed to complete the race just four minutes after me. He was also very satisfied with his final results.

The post-race event was full of fruit, isotonic drinks, water bottles, snacks and gifts. The world of running seemed even more incredible to me, and there I decided something that I still do to this day…

This was only my first race!

MY DIET

When I decided to write this book, it was mainly due to the growing interest of friends and acquaintances in how I managed to lose so much weight (35 kg) in such little time (about five months). In order to reach that goal, I had to change many aspects of my life, such as my diet.

I have always eaten regular food portions, and in my view, I enjoyed simple food – the good old Brazilian "rice, beans, beef and chips." I was never one for dainties such as savoury snacks, hamburgers, cookies and chocolates – I have had to throw away mouldy chocolate bars for lack of eating. My problem has always been lunchtime. Even during my teenage years, I have always eaten too much; my portions would weigh 850 grams and were joined by juices and soft drinks. I always had heavy breakfasts, with eggs, bread, juices and milk. My mother has always insisted that her children did sports, so I have always exercised from a young age. I went swimming, I did athletics, I played basketball and football, I did taekwondo and so on. I have never been fat and I have always eaten regularly. It was hard for me to refuse any kind of food, be it beef, pork, chicken or fish. Although I ate large quantities of a little bit of everything, I also did a lot of sports, so I could always maintain a steady weight.

In 2005, when I was 31 years old, I passed a contest for São Paulo's Civil Police. I used to live with my brother in a ranch in Ubatuba, so I was used to hard work, as well as cycling every time I wanted to go to the city. All that effort kept my weight steady. When I went to the Police Academy, I kept eating as much as before, but I stopped exercising. In little more than a year, I went from 77 kilos to 86 kilos. I did not worry then, since I had the (wrong) impression that I could lose that excessive weight whenever I wanted. I quickly went from

86 kg to 100 kg. I could not lose weight from the moment that I hit the three-digit mark.

I had the following diet: I would have a big glass of orange juice, scrambled eggs, bread with processed meats, milk chocolate, fruit and black coffee for breakfast. I would eat salad, rice, beans, any kind of meat and any sides for lunch. At night I usually ate sandwiches and had soft drinks. Extravagant food such as pizza, McDonald's meals, ice-cream, barbecues and beer were not uncommon.

In those years (around 2007), I also started dating and attending University after work. I would wake up early, work at the police station from 9 am to 7 pm, go straight to class and leave at 11 pm. On the weekends, I would go on dates or spend time with my parents. When I was dating, I used to go out to eat or to the food court in a shopping centre. When I was home, I would devour my mother's cooking and I'd eat candy from our cupboards. I did not care about my weight then, and it reached 117 kilos.

I didn't have time to exercise, nor did I want to. I was working, studying and dating. Every part of my life seemed good, so I had that feeling that all was well. My then girlfriend used to say that I needed to take care of myself. We enrolled in a gym for a month but then gave up.

In 2011 when I was married and still working at the Police Department, I got scared when my blood pressure reached 210/190 mm Hg. I was sent to the hospital and I started taking pills to control it. My wife, my mother and my friends at work started monitoring my eating habits and pressuring me into taking care of myself. I started exercising in my apartment building's gym before going to work. I managed to lose a few kilos with a little effort, but I was still far from being healthy nor out of peril. I graduated in Law in 2012 and left the police force to work as a lawyer. I stopped exercising, since I had to start working earlier in my new job. I worked for that company until 2013. I moved back to Ubatuba in March 2013, and when I got there I was weighing 107 kilos and had a sedentary lifestyle.

My brother was setting up a restaurant and he asked me to partner up with him. I had been wanting to return to Ubatuba for a while, since my life in Sao Paulo no longer satisfied me and I wanted to provide my wife with a better quality of life. At that time, I also wanted to have a child, so I thought it would be better for him/her not to grow up in an apartment. My idea of moving back to Ubatuba comprised a better life and a quieter place to raise a family. I didn't think twice: I took up my brother's offer and returned to Ubatuba (I moved back to our ranch), but I had to leave my wife in Sao Paulo.

After living in Ubatuba for a year and a half, with our restaurant set up and working from nine in the morning to our last customer – which was up to two in the morning on weekends – I ended up losing some weight, since I walked a lot and cycled, but I was still on the verge of one hundred kilos and I did not have any workout routine. I felt sick in the restaurant twice, but I was not taken to the hospital. My diet was terrible, even though I now worked in a restaurant. My daily schedule was messes up and I worked more than what I used to work in São Paulo, since I worked two shifts in the restaurant.

I got divorced in September 2014 and that was when I hit rock bottom, since in addition to not caring about my health, I also did not care about my looks. I was sure that it couldn't get worse and even if it did, I did not care. When I had my epiphany and was willing to change my negligent situation, I had to change many things, and one of them was indeed difficult... my diet.

For those who want to lose weight, having an adequate diet is as important as being active. After more than a year of getting to know my body and learning how to lose weight, I can say that only changing one's diet is *not* enough to lose weight. I dare say that only exercising is also not enough to lose excessive weight. In order to do so adequately, the best you can do is to control your diet in addition to doing regular exercise.

It is very hard to talk about eating habits, since that is something very personal to me. Everyone to his taste. Altering one's diet is akin to altering one's mood. We all like eating well, so being forced to it tasteless foods or giving up eating our favourite foods causes all kinds of side effects, such as annoyance, mood swings, insomnia and even depression.

When I was losing weight, one of the most widely asked question was: "How did you manage to lose so much weight?" I always told them: "In order to lose weight, one has to make sacrifices." This is true. Not a single diet will work if you are not willing to make sacrifices.

When I wanted to lose weight, I looked for a method with which I'd get quick results without effort. I learned that no such method exists. There is no such thing as weight loss without effort. One must be disciplined to reach their goals. I tried the moon diet, the blood type diet, the carbohydrate diet, the notes diet, the dots diet, the juices diet, the teas diet... I tried them all, indeed. I even got good results in some of them, but always as a result of hard work.

I never liked mathematics, but it has followed, or persecuted me all my life. When I studied Computer Science in university, I found that its basic courses are all science-based, and so I had to study matrixes, vector trigonometry, calculus and physics. Not surprisingly, I dropped out. When I started law school, I came across labour legal calculations and child support payments. After opening my restaurant, I had to deal with math again, this time in accounting spreadsheets and stock-taking. In fact, math appeared in my life again when I started losing weight. Allow me to explain.

Every diet that includes calorie reduction is effective for weight loss. In other words, remember that our bodies need an energy source to move or to act. Let us consider that this energy source are calories. We need energy to do our daily activities, such as working, tidying the house, going to the gym, and even sleeping. That energy is the calorie that we get from food. Every food has its amount of calories, be it even more or less calories. Therefore, we need a certain amount of calories a day to perform our daily tasks. By comparison, it is as if our bodies were cars and depending on how much fuel we had, our engine would run more or less. When there is no more fuel, the car has to get it from the reserve gasoline tank. As a result, we can say that our bodies need a certain calorie consumption to execute its daily functions. When you consume an amount of calories that is inferior to what you need, your body will get energy from your reserves, that is, fats. However, when you consume more calories than necessary, your body will store the excessive calories, which then become fat, like those on our waists. I then realised the importance of maths on my life. Losing weight is indeed an exact science. The magic formula for losing weight is simple:

The weight loss theorem is: SPENDING > CONSUMING. You have to spend more than you consume. That is the secret and the path to success. For instance, if someone spends 1,000 calories on a day, but consumes 999 calories, they will lose weight, even if takes eighty years.

Nowadays, with the advent of internet, it's much easier to find out how many calories we need. There are websites with tables that calculate spending per exercise, based on your gender, age and weight. It is possible to find out even how much energy you spend when you are asleep. This is extremely important to know before starting any diet. After all, how will you know how much you need to consume if you still do not know how much energy you spend? You can and must get the information regarding how many calories your body needs on a daily basis, through research or with professional help.

In the introduction to this book, I mentioned that I have no formal education in health-related fields whatsoever, so what I did was based on deduction, reading, studying and self-awareness – a trial and error process. What I managed to do worked out for me, for my body and for the goal I'd set. This is not to say that this method will work for you and that you must try it out; on the contrary, I am here just to tell you what I did. If you wish to follow your steps, please be advised that you are on your own and that my body is different from yours, and so is my metabolism, my routine and my eating habits. What worked out for me might not work out for you.

When I started working out, I did not change my diet. My daily one-hour walks caused me to lose some weight, but that wasn't what I wanted. I could not lose weight just by exercising, no matter how intense my work outs got. I was losing weight slowly and that was very discouraging. It was only when I realised that I must change my diet that I got better results. I was reluctant to change my diet, since I love eating and I'd have to give up something I enjoyed so much if I really wanted to change my looks.

I still did not know what I should eat nor the quantity I had to ingest to achieve my goals. It took me weeks of trial and error to find out a meal plan that I could follow without too much effort. During my first few weeks of walking, I read a lot about dieting and combining meal plans. I would buy health magazines that contained meal plans and recipes for diets. However, the issue of cost is never addressed – if you follow the recipes from those magazines and wish to follow their meal plans, which are prepared by celebrities' nutritionists, be prepared to spend a lot of money on your credit card. Although you will eat delicious food, you will have to splurge. Indeed, dieting with tasty ingredients, diet and imported products will cost you an arm and a leg and will make you give up, and thus you will feel like a loser. A good diet is created with daily ingredients, which can be found at any self-service restaurant. It is vital to keep in mind that your diet must be based on foods that you are used to eating; with that, it will be much easier to face that challenge.

The first thing I did when I decided to lose weight was to discover my daily calorie expenditure. After searching through many tables, I found that my body needed a daily calorie intake of 3,200 calories. I should make it clear that such an amount was based on my gender, weight, age, physical activity practice and moments of rest. Now that I knew that my daily intake was of 3,200 calories, I knew that I could follow any diet whose total consumption was less than that amount of calories.

I chose to follow a diet in which I could consume a thousand calories at the most, which would cause a difference of 2,000 calories per day, which, as I later found out, meant 200 grams a day. Now that I knew how many calories I could consume every day, I got a calorie chart of popular foods and created a meal plan for each of my meals.

To clarify, a Big Mac has 500 calories, a medium drink has 200 calories and medium fries have around 300 calories. Therefore, a lunch at McDonald's was enough to reach my daily calorie consumption limit. With that in mind, I understood that I could eat anything, even a McDonald's meal, but that would be my only meal of the day. It would be smarter to try and distribute all those calories in at least three meals throughout my day. The most difficult part of creating a meal plan is the daily calorie limit. I also created a rule: "Any calories left to consume were noncumulative. These calories would not be available on to the next day."

I used to carry around a food calorie table which I'd found on the internet. I would check it all the time to see how many calories a cup of coffee had, as well as in a slice of melon, a slice of cheese, and so on – I'd check the calories of every single food I'd put in my mouth. Although it may seem like an insane thing to do, everyone does this. After a while, I got used to the calories and I knew how many portions I could eat of any given food. My diet consisted of 800 to 1,100 calories a day. Once a month, I'd allow myself to eat some delicacies – my "extravagance day".

This was my meal plan during the months in which I lost weight the most:

Breakfast: One piece of fruit, a glass of any sugar-freejuice or sugar-free tea.

Lunch: Lettuce salad, corn, peas, tomatoes, onions, cucumbers, heart-of-palms, carrots and any 200 grams steak (beef, pork, fish or chicken)

Dinner: One carrot, orange and honey yogurt, or just a honey yogurt.

Snack: Fruit.

I wouldn't eat any fried food, delicacies, breads, snacks, pasta nor dessert. When I wanted to eat any of those things, I'd eat it on my monthly extravagance day or I ate a small portion of it and later made up for it in any other meals.

While it isn't good to always eat the same thing, the easiest part of following a diet is to eat food that is readily available. There is no use in putting dried dates in your snack if you only buy it once a year. It is best not to get too creative. Anyone can make a good lettuce, tomato and onion salad. If you are a bit more creative, mix some cooked vegetables on your salad and that's it – however, you can change salad dressings. I needn't tell you to remove mayonnaise-based dressings from your diet, but you can use olive oil, lemons, vinegar, salt, soy sauce, balsamic and so on are good options. Furthermore, don't skip the steak, since eating a 200-250 grams steak will be good for your health. For instance, you could eat a medium top sirloin or a grilled half-chicken breast, as well as pork chop, grilled pork ham, or perhaps a grilled hake steak. I am sure that exaggerating in meat consumption won't be bad for your health.

My lunch was composed of a medium salad bowl and a 200 grams steak. When I started dieting, I'd put the salad on a platter, I'd put the stake on a plate and I would use another plate to eat, thus eating slowly. When I got used to it, though, I'd chop my salad and grate the vegetables, then use soy sauce and olive oil dressing. As for the steak, I'd chop it up and fry it, then add it to the mixture. It was truly akin to a swamp in its appearance, but I that much food would satisfy me completely. The bright side of eating salad is that you can eat as much as you want. I ate huge portions of salad until I was bloated, and sometimes I had to force myself to eat the steak. After reaching your ideal weight, you will be able to eat more calories and you will thus change your meal plan.

This is why it is vital to include foods that you can eat and that you are used to eating in your meal plan. I remember that I had to eat half a papaya with fax seeds in one of the diets I tried, and I didn't like it. It was hard to swallow and it was hard to eliminate, so do not force yourself to eat what you don't like. It is never going to work.

I chose foods that I could eat for weeks on end. While they were not delicious, they would help me lose weight. My salad was, then, composed of all the ingredients I mentioned. Please note that dieting is not cheap and that vegetables must be bought every other day. A head of lettuce lasts three days at the most, while canned corn lasts for four meals. A pickled heart-of-palm lasted six meals, while I used a carrot, one Japanese cucumber, 1/3 of an onion and a whole tomato per meal. A kilo of top sirloin lasted four or five meals, and so did most meats.

You must have heard that one must have self-control in order to start dieting. I believe that eating is a need and an addiction – it is a need when we are not dieting, and it becomes an addiction when we have to stop eating delicious foods. From an addict's point of view, we must face abstinence from delicious foods in the same way that an alcoholic faces abstinence from alcohol. I own a restaurant that serves feijoada, rabada[2] and many other dishes that I love. Imagine how it was for me to be tempted by the aromas and by customers savouring good food. Indeed, it takes a lot of self-control not to devour these foods. I have had to leave the restaurant to take a break, in order to lessen my desperation and my willingness to throw everything out of the window and devour the crunchy chips covered in garlic, which is one of my favourite dishes. Thus, I urge you *not to test yourself!* Try to avoid going to places where your resistance and self-control will be put to the test – in the beginning, skip self-service restaurants. Do not go

---

[2]Feijoada and rabada are popular, traditional Brazilian dishes. (T.N.)

to the supermarket when hungry. Do not attend children's parties, filled to the brim with fried snacks and sweets. It is helpful to leave home stuffed only with the food you planned to eat. As I own restaurant, there was no escaping the temptation. My self-control was tested to the point of exhaustion – the only thing worse than seeing those dishes and smelling the aromas was to see people feasting on them. The key word here is *focus*!

Food deprivation is and always will be complicated, but one must think that mankind was not made to eat fried food, pasta, chocolates nor many other delicacies. Humans are omnivores by nature – the fact that we have canines and molars means something. Our basic diet can and should be comprised of fruit, vegetables and meats. No one will suffer by not eating salty pastries nor McDonald's meals. One must *focus* in what will change their body in a healthy way.

My grandfather used to say the following: "There are no fat men in concentration camps." I know this sounds awful, but it is partially true – lack of food will make you lose a lot of weight, but in a bad way. It is best to lose weight while being healthy. I didn't get sick at all when I was losing weight. When starting a diet, many people tend to cut out good things and bad things from their meal plans. As a result, they get weak, underfed and even anaemic. In order to avoid that, it is important to remember that our bodies need vitamins, proteins, fibres, mineral salts and carbohydrates, besides many other chemical compounds that I will not mention. If such substances are ingested in the right way, there is no way to get weak nor sick. Therefore, I started planning my diet based on salad (vitamins and fibres), fruit (sugar and vitamins) and meat (proteins). You must be asking yourself: *What about carbohydrates?* Well, carbohydrates are the main source of energy for our bodies, and I had a lot of them in my belly, legs, buttocks, neck area, and in my whole body – those were my energy reserves. Thus, I removed them from my diet, although I would end up ingesting some of them on vegetables, even though I didn't need them, since I just wanted my body to burn those I already had by using them as its main energy source. I know this must sound like gibberish to you, so allow me to explain.

Imagine the following situation: two people – one of them is obese and sedentary, while the other person is athletic and does not have much fat in their body. Place them on a deserted island without food. Who do you think will survive for longer? If you chose the athletic person, you are absolutely wrong. The athletic person does not have any fat reserves and muscles demand a lot of energy, hence they would soon get weak, dehydrate and perish. The fat person, on the other hand, has a many fat reserves, which their body will consumewhen necessary. That was my train of thought: my body would need to consume all my fat reserves. In order to do that, I needed to keep my body healthy, thus providing it with all the vitamins, fibres and proteins that it needed, excluding carbohydrates, which it would have to get from my fat reserves. This is why I stopped eating pasta, fried food and anything else that contained huge quantities of carbohydrates. The amount of carbohydrates I consumed when eating vegetables was not enough to make a difference. Funnily enough, most high-calorie foods have starch and sugars.

In addition, sugar was a problem. When consulting calorie tables for the dishes I used to eat, I noticed that all industrialised products had very high levels of sugar, so I stopped eating dessert. I started eating more sugar-free or diet food, like soft drinks and juice, as well as industrialised foods. I would avoid eating patisserie sweets such as cookies and so on. However, I did not stop putting sugar in my coffee, since I'd rather not drink coffee at all than addsweetenersor drink plain black coffee.

It is important to remember that this cutting-out-of-my-diet strategy was conducted gradually, not all at once. When I started my walking workouts, I would eat normally, without changing my diet, and thus I lost those five kilos. After that, I reduced my food portions by half, which resulted in more weight loss. The next step was to exercise more, which helped me lose even more weight. Finally, I started cutting out food from my diet until I reached my ideal meal plan, as previously mentioned. This process took a couple of months and I believe that I probably would not have achieved such good results if I had started cutting out food as soon as I had begun walking, since I would not have been able to control my diet. Here is another tip – you should cut out food from your diet in a gradual manner. In order to better understand this, imagine the following: when I started dieting, I needed to ingest 3,200 calories to maintain my weight. In order to lose weight, I needed to reduce my daily calorie intake until I consumed 1,000 calories a day, which I did until I reached my ideal weight.The thinner one is, the less calories they will need – so if I needed 2,800 calories a day instead of 3,200 calories to maintain my weight, my diet should be reduced in order for it to have the same impact on my body.

Never stop focusing on your goal, on your ideal weight and especially on the body that you want to see in your reflection. Whenever you feel hungry, try to imagine yourself happy, on your ideal weight, healthy. This will help you control your food cravings.

It is probably much harder to stop eating things we love than getting up at five in the morning to walk on a rainy day, *but there is no other way*. There is no weight loss if you keep eating chocolate, snacks and drinking litres of soft drinks every day. You *will* have to stop drinking beer, caipirinha[34] and having barbecues for a while and there will be no pizzas, pastries nor coffee.

I guarantee that giving up those delicacies will have extremely positive consequences for your body and life.

---

[3]Caipirinha: a typical Brazilian cocktail made with cachaça, sugar, and lime. There are many variations on the fruit and alcoholic beverages used – common variations include strawberries, tangerines, lemons, passion fruit, vodka, sake, etc.
[4] Cachaça is a traditional Brazilian distilled spirit made from fermented sugar cane juice.

MY FIRST HALF-MARATHON

I had been running for six months. I had already participated in three races: the "Soldado Paulino" 10 km race, the "Speedo Run" race in São Paulo, which was also a 10 km race, and the "Physical Educator Day Race", a 7 km race which was promoted by one of Ubatuba's gyms.

When I was about to sign up for my fourth race – at this point, my workouts were planned according to upcoming races – I came across a race that was divided in three parts (categories). It was composed of a five kilometre walk, a ten kilometre race and a half-marathon of twenty-one kilometres. My brother was visiting on that day, and when I told him about this race, he asked me whether I'd participate on the half-marathon. I told him no, that I wasn't able to do it. He then asked me: "Until when are you going to run these little ten kilometre races?" That bugged me. Is running ten kilometres so bad to the point of being referred to as "little races"?

We have a popular saying among runners: "It doesn't matter how much you run, just run". I have always focused on my elapsed time when exercising, not on how many kilometres I run, since distance is a consequence of preparation. I increased my distance depending on whether I needed to run for an hour, but I was able to cover fifteen kilometres almost daily. Was it time to face bigger challenges? Was I ready to take the next step or to add seven kilometres to my workouts? Such questions would not leave me alone. My runs were more than*little races*.

With that in mind, I found on the internet that only two races with less than twenty-one kilometres had national recognition. One of them is the Volta da Pampulha, which took place in Belo Horizonte, Minas Gerais[5] and consisted of running around the Pampulha Lake. The other one is the Saint

---

[5] Belo Horizonte is the capital city of the state of Minas Gerais in south-eastern Brazil. The Pampulha is an administrative region of Belo Horizonte and is divided into nine districts or neighbourhoods. It has an artificial lake in its centre, known as the Pampulha Lake, one of the city's main tourist attractions.

Silvester Road Race[6], which is held yearly in São Paulo on December 31 and its course is 15 km long. Since it is so prestigious, I believe that it needs no introduction. Apart from these two races, other prestigious races are half-marathons and marathons. The most prestigious half-marathons of Brazil are the Rio Half-Marathon and the São Paulo International Marathon, which have elite athletes and Olympicmedallists among its participants. In addition, these are important international events which are usually shown on television. The world's six largest and most renowned marathons consist of The Abbott World Marathon Majors, whose races take place in Tokyo, Boston, London, Berlin, Chicago and New York City.

The more I learned about marathons, the more excited I got. How in the world had I never paid attention to any of this? These events were very well-produced and the athletes seemed to be involved in a positive environment. Thus, I started watching new and old races from all over the world on YouTube, and I also started reading books and magazines about marathons. After reading about marathons and half-marathons, I was inclined to signing up for the next race, and despite the long-distance run, I remembered what my brother said and thus signed up for the half-marathon.

---

[6] This is the oldest and most prestigious street race in Brazil.

I would have run twenty-one kilometres, something that I had never thought possible. Only a few months prior, I was sitting on my couch, eating all sorts of junk food and watching the same film for the thousandth time... gaining weight. In that time, I never imagined that I would be able to run a kilometre, let alone a half-marathon. I needn't mention how proud I was of this achievement, but the idea of running a half-marathon was a bit scary, since I was still an amateur athlete. In fact, covering twenty-one kilometres meant running for at least two hours on an average pace. Could I do it?

I had just paid the fee. When I received the email confirming my registration, I felt like I was on a roller coaster, with no turning back. Suddenly, it seemed that the date of the race was approaching, although there were still three months left. I marked the date on my calendar: October 25. 2015... the day of my first half-marathon!

I had almost three months to prepare for the race. At this point, I weighed 75 kilos. My diet was normal again, but I'd eat only small portions of foods like rice, beans, potatoes, pasta, bread and some fried food, since I was concerned about maintaining my weight. I avoided junk food in order to preserve my health rather than because of its high-calorie contents. I ate little bit of everything, but I was still careful about meal times and calorie consumption.

I have previously mentioned the relevance of getting to know one's body and how to read its signs. I learned in the worst possible way that I couldn't eat late in the evening and that I had to be very careful about what I ate if I had to train on the next day, since some kinds of food give me cramps while running – to the point of putting an end to my workout sessions. I cannot eat pasta, sauces, grains nor fried food on the night before working out. This is something I learned by observing my body. In the beginning, I used to think that I was not breathing correctly, but I later realised it was gas, so I came to the conclusion that the food I ate on the day before could not ferment inside my body or I'd get cramps. In order to solve this problem, I would have to eat hours before going to bed so that the foo would be digested, or I could eat light foods such as yogurts, processed meats or fruit, or I could go to the toilet before working out. As a result, my cramps disappeared.

I started preparing for the upcoming half-marathon by creating a workout spreadsheet. I had no knowledge of professional preparation for running, nor did I have any money to enrol in a gym nor to hire a personal trainer. My idea was simple, however: I had to cover a longer distance than the distance of the half-marathon one month before the event.I would feel confident enough to finish the race if I managed to cover twenty-five kilometres, and the only way to do that was to gradually increase my running distance during my work outs.

The first thing I did was to understand what twenty-five kilometreswere. I created various twenty-one kilometres routes on Google Maps. However, for you to have an idea, this was like completing the route from my house to the Caisão of Ubatuba three times. I wasn't going to take this route again, since running laps is very boring to me and I would prefer to create a new route. I wanted to avoid unnecessary slopes when creating my routes, so I realised that twenty-one kilometres was a long distance indeed. I could go from my house to Itamambuca beach, which was sixteen kilometres away, or I could go past the Rio Escuro neighbourhood. In Sao Paulo, I could go from my parents' house in Jardim Bonfiglioli[7] to the nearby city of Cotia.

I believe that the most important factor to be taken into account when creating a route, especially long routes, is that it ends on your doorstep. However, I only realised that

---

[7] Jardim Bonfiglioli is a district in the Butantã neighbourhood, located in the west zone of the city of São Paulo.

when I had to take a bus home after a thirty-four kilometre run. I had decided to go to the nearby city of Caraguatatuba in one of my longer routes as part of my marathon training. I had to wait for the bus for hours while tired, sweaty, hungry, thirsty, and a long way from Ubatuba – it took me hours to get home on that day. I should have taken the bus to Caraguatatuba and run back home.

In other words, I suggest that you finish your workout route on your doorstep or in front of your car. The point is that by the time your training session is over, you will be able to relax at home or on the car on your way home. This is very important and must be thought about in a thorough manner when you decide to increase your running time and distance. I have had to return home by foot whilst exhausted or on muscle cramps because I had chosen a bad route. Keep in mind that you should be safe when you finish your workout in the sense that you should be able to eat, drink, relax or at the very least you should be in an urban area.

Most of the routes I chose involved the Rio-Santos highway, which goes through Ubatuba. I was a bit scared of running on that highway because it is quite dangerous to run on a winding road early in the morning, when there is little to no visibility. Furthermore, I would have to share the roadside with pedestrians, cyclists, and bus drivers that stop along the highway, not to mention drivers driving past at least sixty kilometres per hour. I had to think about and plan ahead. Therefore, I decided to take a route similar to the one I covered on my daily workouts. By that time, I was already used to covering fifteen kilometres between Perequê-Açubeach to the Caisão and back, so I only had to add six kilometres to the route. I decided to add the Praia Grande beach. I would now leave home having the end of Perequê-Açu as a destination, then I would return in the direction of the Caisão; on the roundabout at the end of the Itaguá Avenue (Leovigildo Dias Vieira Avenue), I'd turn right on Capitão Felipe Avenue on my way to Rio-Santos. I would cover a distance of three-hundred metres on Rio-Santos, then I would enter the street on the shore of Praia Grande and run to its very end, on the beginning of the lookout slope. After that, I would return to the Itaguá Avenue, then I would return to the Caisão, then I would be home. This route had twenty-one kilometres just like I wanted.

Now that I was a participant in a half-marathon, getting up in the morning had a new meaning. My daily workout did become professional training and I was more careful about my diet, avoiding desserts and late night snacks. I would run up to sixty kilometres a week and walk briskly on the boardwalk by the seashore on Sunday afternoons. After two weeks of training, in a Wednesday in August, I decided that it was time to try running twenty-five kilometres. I wanted to test myself, so I scheduled that long run for the next Sunday.

I started preparing for that long run. I worked out normally on Thursday and Friday and even tried harder on the last few kilometres. I monitored my diet with care and had no surprises. I thought that bringing water with me was not necessary, since I would exercise for only forty minutes longer than usual. On that Sunday, I woke up excitedly, before my alarm rang. I felt confident when I looked at myself in the mirror before leaving. I had never been better. I put on shorts, socks, running shoes and a very bright orange t-shirt. Since I was going to run on the edge of the highway for a while, I had better be visible. It was still dark when I left home. The day was very cold, cloudy and humid. I stretched, started my stopwatch and started running.

I listened to calm, rhythmic songs on my way to Perequê-Açu beach. I ran calmly, without worrying about my elapsed time. I ran to the edge of the beach and returned, then I reached the roundabout in the end of Itaguá Avenue. The sun was rising when I entered Capitão Felipe Avenue and the cloudy sky cleared, and when I arrived in Praia Grande beach on my thirteenth kilometre, the sun appeared. When I had finished running in Praia Grande and was near the highway, the sun shone brightly and I was exhausted. I had run sixteen kilometres and my legs faltered when I climbed the ramp to enter Rio-Santos. That drew my attention as I felt my right leg falter, as if my knee bended involuntarily. I pressed on, though.

I had already run seventeen kilometres and few hundred metres and I was reaching the Capitão Felipe Avenue when it happened. The best way to describe it is the following: "Imagine burying an incandescent knitting needle in your thigh." I felt that prick on my right leg, it immediately went stiff and burned. It hurt and burned at the same time, like being stung by a giant bee. It hurt; *it hurt a lot*! A tear fell from my eye. In that moment, I stopped, put my hand on my leg and knelt, bowing to my carelessness. I was also bowing to my lack of humility, to the fact that I was not ready yet and that I had been exaggerating on the last few weeks. The Gods of running taught me in that moment the definition of insurmountable object. I remained in that position for a few minutes as I cursed at myself. I walked home plodding on my way there.

As a result of my carelessness, I did not run for two weeks. I felt a lot of pain on my right thigh every time I moved for two weeks, even simple movements such as climbing the stairs or getting up from the couch. Whatever happened on that day had hurt my thigh. On the second of week of rest, the pain diminished, then subsided on the third week. During my recovery period, I massaged my thigh and pressed a cold compress on it. I avoided forcing my leg and I started going to work by car, and I also tried to sit down at work and stretch out my legs. Fortunately, the pain disappeared a month after that fateful day. However, with that injury, I learned how necessary it was to respect my body's limits. No one is Superman. If you exaggerate, your body will respond, and perhaps you will learn the hard the way, like I did.

After a month without exercise, some things changed. I realised that I gained four kilos and now weighed 79 kilos. I was lazy, my house was messy again, I went back to eating late night snacks, going to bed late and thus waking up late. I needed to get back into working out! Now that the race was only six weeks away, I had to lose weight and get back into my old routine. One day after work I put on my running shoes and went for a run on the boardwalk to "test" my thigh. I began by walking on a briskly pace for a kilometre, then ran faster for another kilometre. I walked for a while, then walked briskly again, then sprinted. There was no pain. I thought I had recovered, so I ran back my home on my regular pace. I was happy.

I now needed to recover all the time lost, starting by losing weight again. Since I feared injuring myself again, I decided to run the race weighing 72 kg, so that I would not pressure my muscles. I would have a little over a month to lose 7 kg. I went back to dieting.

I went back to working out and started slowly. On my first workouts, I ran between five and ten kilometres. I only went back to my old workout routine two weeks later, and during that time I controlled my diet and exercised constantly. I paid attention to my right leg, although I had not felt any more pain.

There was just a month left for the race and I felt almost completely recovered. I now worried about not testing myself, which consisted of running a longer distance than the race on a long run. My weekends were almost over and I needed to do that on a free Sunday. A long run workout demands not only time to complete it, but also time for recovering afterwards. I usually sleep after a long-distance run or race. I get home, take a shower, drink plenty of waterand get something to eat, then sleep for a couple of hours. Therefore, I had to find a way to do a long run (a distance that I had never run before) in a Sunday.

I had decided to do my long run three Sundays before the race, since that would give me more than enough time to recover. My goal was just to run twenty-five kilometres in two hours and a half, which was more than enough time to test my resistance and most importantly, my thigh.

During the days that preceded my long run, I was still choosing a route when my friend Zildo Lopes showed up on my restaurant. We talked about many subjects, including running and workouts. Zildo mentioned that he wanted to run on the days that he would be in Ubatuba and asked me whether I had ever run to Vermelha do Norte beach. He convinced me that it was worth a try and he told me that it had only a small slope before reaching the beach. I agreed and invited him to join me on that long run. Just like that, I had a running partner yet again.

I got up very early on that Sunday, put on my workout clothes and took my vitamins along with a glass of sugar-free mate tea. I opted not to take any water with me. Zildo arrived at the agreed time, left his things in my house and we left to stretch. We agreed to meet again in my house in case we got separated. I turned on my music, started my stopwatch and then we started running. We crossed Iperoig and Cruzeiro beaches together. When we reached the Barra dos Pescadores bridge, which gives access to the end of Perequê-Açu beach, I gained some advantage, which had increased to a few blocks by the time we reached the middle of the beach. I ran to the edge of the beach and as there was no street there, I would have to return a few blocks. I met Zildo again, who accompanied me from that point onwards. We ran side by side on a dirt path on the end of Perequê-Açú, which gave us access to Padre Manuel da Nóbrega Avenue, and then to the Rio-Santos highway. We entered the highway and went north. I bypassed Zildo again, who had begun complaining about pain on his foot soles. I kept going and it wasn't long before I climbed the slope and reached the beach. I started returning and found Zildo, who was walking by now. He said that he was in a lot of pain and preferred to return walking. I wanted to accompany him, but he insisted that I focused on my workout. We agreed to meet at my house.

I continued with my workout, now on my way back. I turned in Padre Manoel da Nóbrega Avenue, then to the left on the dirt path to the seashore avenue, then I turned right on this avenue. I crossed the bridge and entered Iperoig Avenue, and then I was running on the boardwalk. I felt good and I was wondering if that route would be enough, since I had forgotten to check the distance on Google Maps. I had been running for an hour and forty minutes, and now I was close to the Ubatuba

Aquarium, which is only three blocks from home. I was tired, but not exhausted – I did not feel any pain in my leg, and I was a bit thirsty. I decided to risk increasing my route by going to the Caisão and then back home. My workout would be forty minutes longer and I would probably run twenty-five kilometres in total.

I kept running on the Itaguá boardwalk, even running past my street, increasing my run metre by metre. I had been running for two hours and now I was thirsty. I regretted not having bought a water bottle when I ran past by some stalls. While on my way to the Caisão, I imagined that if I came across a worker from the ice factory, I would ask them for some water – that was the extent of my thirst. When I reached the ice factory, it was closed. I took a deep breath and pressed on until I reached the Caisão. I stepped on its concrete floor, took a turn and started returning home. When I ran past the boat gas station near the ice factory, I saw a hose attached to a water spurt. I approached and noticed that there was no one there. I held the hose by its tip and turned on the faucet. The water gushed out with intensity and I swallowed mouthful after mouthful of water and I also washed my hair and face. I turned it off and kept running with renewed motivation. I arrived home with two hours and thirty minutes of elapsed time. Zildo was already there, waiting for me. He told me that he felt a very strange pain, which bothered him so much that he couldn't keep running, so he walked back to my house. He said that he would check it out, but he was sure that he would get better soon.

As soon as Zildo left, I took a shower and later checked on my workout data. The first thing I did was to trace the route on Google Maps in order to find out the distance I had just run. After a while, I managed to create the correct route – 24.77 km! That was a fantastic achievement! I was so happy that I did a little dance in front of my computer. I had managed to complete my workout with honours, I was okay, fit and ready for the race. Without pain nor tiredness. Most importantly, I was confident. *Let the 21K come!*

After that long run, I decided that my test was as good as done, so all I had to do now was to stay fit and focus on working out more, with care not to injure myself. At this point, many people already knew about the race and I did not try to hide this information from them – on the contrary, more people knew about it because I talked about it whenever I could.

The remaining weeks passed by quickly and that Saturday arrive – the eve of the race. I was planning to work until around 5 PM and take the bus to São Paulo at 5:30 PM. As usual, my mother would pick me up at the Butantã underground station and we would go home. On that Saturday, I woke up as usual, but stayed in bed for another hour since I would not have to train.I got up, had some coffee and took Vicky for a walk. The day went by fast and the restaurant was busy. As the day ended, I rushed to the bus station and boarded the bus to São Paulo. It had been a good idea to take the bus, since I'd be able to sleep for a few hours. As we had agreed, my mother picked me up on the underground station and took me home. I set out my clothes for the next day, took a shower and turned on every alarm available before going to bed.

I woke up around five in the morning on the day of the race, got ready and packed the things I'd decided to take with me. I drove my mother's car to the starting point of the race, which was near Transamérica Expo Center.[8] I decided to leave early for a number of reasons: I did not know which streets would be closed, nor did I know where to park the car – I might need to park it far away and walk to the starting point, I needed a locker to store my things and I had to find *my* own starting point for the race. That was why I left home an hour

[8]Transamérica Expo Center, also known as Centro de ConvençõesTransamérica ("Transamerica Convention Centre") is a convention centre in Santo Amaro, a neighbourhood in the south zone of São Paulo.

earlier. I was almost at the convention centre when I noticed a crowd heading to the Arena.

I arrived in the convention centre an hour before the start of the race. I left my mother's car in its parking lot, which cost me fifty reais[9], which seemed absurd[10] to me. In my opinion, a race like Athenas, which has quite the expensive registration fee, should provide athletes with their own parking lot or at the very least charge reasonable prices. Unfortunately, that is also the case with race expos, as parking is costly. I wish I could take quality public transportation that would allow me to arrive in time for races or expos, but that is utopian. We do not yet have such a good public transportation system in the country which would allow you to leave your car at home and still be on time for any event. That is how it is, sadly.

I left the car and accompanied the colourful crowd as it made its way towards the Arena. When I am heading to a race, I never worry about knowing the location of the gates or of the starting line, since you can always go with the flow in order to find out. I was amazed by what I saw as soon as I set foot inside the Arena. There were many stalls offering services, showing running equipment and sports supplies. There was a

[9]The Brazilian Real is the country's national currency (BRL).
[10]São Paulo is known for its lack of parking spots and also for its expensive private parking lots.

stage in which fitness instructors were giving exercises and bigphoto panels. In short, a myriad of interesting activities. The environment before and after a race is always contagious and the energy in the air is almost palpable with everyone in a good mood and excited about the race.

I was able to quickly find a locker, where I stored my bag. Now that I only had what I would need for the race, I tried to find my starting point. In bigger races there is a group division just before the start of the race, which is based on each athlete's individual pace. The groups remain divided by tape until the start, so that faster runners will not be hindered by slow runners. I found my starting point and started doing my stretches.

The "Athenas 21K" is a race of the Athenas series, promoted by Iguana Sports. It has three stages throughout the year: the first stage is a 10K race, the second stage is a 15K race, and the third stage is a 21K race. The idea behind it is that the runner attempts to increase his challenge throughout the year. The route consisted of running in Marginal Pinheiros, crossing the river through Ponte Estaiada[11], running a good

---

[11] Ponte Estaiada is a popular name for Octávio Frias de Oliveira Bridge, is a cable-stayed bridge in São Paulo, one of the highlights of the city. It is over the Pinheiros River and it connects Marginal Pinheiros, in the west zone of the city, to Jornalista Roberto Marinho Avenue, in the south zone.

stretch on the opposite bank of the river and then we would return to the start. In aerial view, we would run in an "H" shape using the bridge, which was the main attraction of the course. I enjoy running past places which I can only access by car, so Ponte Estaida as well as Marginal Pinheiros were such places to me.

As soon as the race started, I set my stopwatch and crossed the start gate. I was excited, but also nervous. I had not planned nor trained any strategy, so I'd only try to finish the course on my usual time, without increasing nor diminishing it. We ran a good stretch in Marginal Pinheiros until we reached the access to the bridge. I did not imagine, nor do drivers normally notice, how long and steep that slope is. That climb took my breath away and my pace diminished, but the good part is that going down was easy and it allowed me to take a deep breath and relax my muscles. We returned and entered the bridge again after a few hundred metres, but this time we crossed the river. This time, climbing that slope was easier. I ran a few more kilometres on the opposite bank of the river and I still was not thirsty. The weather was cold and humid, which was helpful. I entered the bridge once again and crossed the river.

After running fifteen kilometres, I felt that my body was hot, so I grabbed a plastic cup of water, filled my mouth with it, gargled and spat it, since I just wanted to remove that salty taste of my mouth. I dropped the rest on my head, which relieved the heat. I started feeling tired when there were two kilometres left for the race to end. I felt a sharp pain on my thigh, but that did not make me stop.

When I reached the 20K sign, one of the race monitors shouted: "Come on! You made it all the way here, just go and finish the race!" That was like a lion's roar to my ears. I turned up the volume on my iPhone and ran faster. I could now see the spectators and the finish gate at the end of the corridor. In that moment I needn't have legs, breath nor body. The thrill of finishing a race is what carries you to the finish line. I did not feel any pain nor exhaustion, my thigh did not hurt anymore and I had stopped worrying about it, so everything seemed perfect. It is funny that, when you are on the finish line, the runners that run past you greet you, and compliment other runners, congratulating each other for finishing the race. We were all going through the same challenge, so everyone knows what you have been through, since they also have, which is very good.

I collected two Gatorades – I had not drunk anything during the race – as well as my post-race snack, an apple and my longed-for medal. It was the biggest one yet, and it was golden, with a fire carved on it, representing the completion of my first half-marathon. I made my way to the main Arena, where the massage and sports equipment stalls and lockers were located, since I had to recover my bag.

The production of such events is indeed interesting, since one gets many gifts, food, discount coupons and so much more. I strolled for a bit, then took the car and went home. As I drove past Marginal Pinheiros, I could see some runners finishing the race, which brought a smile to my face. I gifted myself a used Garmin Forerunners 220. *First half-marathon...mission accomplished*!

ACCESSORIES

One of the reasons why I started walking and then running is the fact that it is a cheap exercise. You do not need anything other than shorts and a t-shirt to begin working out.

I remember that I would wear the sneakers that I had at the time. I used to wear Nike Shox, which are not great for walking nor running, and also Nike Flex Experience RN3. I had received those Nike RN3 as a birthday present the year before I started dieting, since I already wanted to work out back then. It took me another six months to *start* walking, and in the meantime I wore the sneakers almost daily, which wore it out a bit. These were good, cheap sneakers to start walking, since its soles were made of a material similar to EVA.

Needless to say, not all sneakers are great for running or walking, so it is vital to choose adequate sneakers for this type of exercise. In fact, wearing the wrong type of sneakers can cause serious injuries, so if you intend to buy sneakers, it is best to do your research and ask the retail worker whether the sneakers you wish to buy are adequate for walking or running. I suggest that you do not spend too much money on your first sneakers, since you might give up and thus lose that money, especially because running shoes are not cheap.

I bought my first running shoes when I registered for my first 10K race. I bought months in advance of the race since I wanted to try them out and one should *never* wear new equipment for the first time on a race. I must emphasise that no equipment should be wore for the first time on a race: new running shoes can cause blisters or sore feet, new clothes can cause chafing and new dietary supplements can cause nausea. *Everything* you want to wear on the day of the race *must* be tested before. I do not even wear the t-shirts that are given out at races for two reasons: I do not know what fabric they are made of and whether it may cause chafing or allergies, and these t-shirts tend to release dye and may streak shorts and underwear in bright colours. I usually wear those t-shirts on my workouts or even on my daily routine after thoroughly washing them.

I never had many running shoes since I believe that "if it isn't broke, don't fix it." I chose my running shoes and I always kept the same brand and model. Every time I buy new running shoes, I start wearing the old ones as regular sneakers.

My running shoes usually last four to five months. According to manufacturers, these shoes last around 500 kilometres (which is less than the distance I run in five months). After those months, the running shoes are still good, but the soles are a bit worn, so they can be wore on a daily basis. When I buy new ones, the old ones become daily-use sneakers and I discard my regular sneakers. There are many brands and models of running shoes, which fit all tastes and categories. I advise you to buy comfortable, cushioned running shoes, especially if you are overweight. When your body is used to running, then you can opt for running shoes that are more specific for your preferences. For instance, if you prefer short distance runs, you can buy running shoes with less cushioning. If you prefer long distance runs, choose cushioned running shoes.

It is vital to try on your running shoes before buying them, so you can go to a store and ask shopkeepers for help. Tell them what type of exercise you intend to do and they will show you many options, as in brand, colours, soles, cushioning, etc.

Life has taught me a rule that I consider very accurate: "Not everything that is expensive is good, but everything good is expensive." I am mentioning this because there is a good explanation why famous brands are the most expensive ones. I have never been affluent and when I started working out one of my intentions was to lose weight without having to spend a lot of money, also because I did not have much to spend. I bought workout clothes in a sports equipment store, from a brand that was sold exclusively at this store. It was probably second-hand, since the price difference was huge when compared to famous brands – as I wanted to spend as little money as possible, I chose to buy three "second-hand" clothes instead of one piece of clothing from a famous brand. *What a stupid thing to do!* Those t-shirts were good enough for my walks, but it didn't take long for chafing to appear after I started running farther. That was when I noticed the poor stitching and poorly-made labels. In more than one occasion I could not finish my workout due to chafing caused by stitching. Unfortunately, after refusing to do so, I started spending money on gym wear from famous brands. I started by buying new workout clothes for every race I registered for. Nowadays I only wear shorts, t-shirts, hats and running shoes from famous sports brands. As a result, I never had problems with chafing nor allergies again.

There is a difference between cheap second-hand clothes and expensive clothes from famous brands, and one only notices it after running for a couple of hours. Any t-shirt, even that one picturing your candidate that is running for municipal elections is adequate for walking and running for a few kilometres, but when you for four hours, I guarantee that that t-shirt will hurt your body. At the very least, you will probably face chafing and bleeding nipples by the end of the race.

The most common thing that most people do when they start running is to download an app to monitor their workout. It is interesting to do so, since one can measure their workout times, how many calories were lost, determine pacing and even share the route and exercise with friends on social media (which I think is good, since one will receive a lot of support in response). There are many apps that monitor workouts. All of them have mostly the same resources, so I recommend that you use the one that you like best. I used to use the Nike app. Nowadays, I use Nike, Strava, Garmin, etc.

I believe it is important for you to have your activities stored in some way, since it will be interesting for you to compare and notice your improvement. The mobile phone app stores *all* of it! I have *all* activities I have ever done stored in my apps, from my first walk to this morning's workout. I enjoy comparing my paces from a year ago, review routes and times on certain routes, and any monitoring app will give you with that possibility.

You will surely download one of these apps to your mobile phone along with a big playlist to listen to music while working out, right? I run whilst listening to music, since that helps me relax. I believe that the run gets a lot more fun and less tiring, but have you ever seen a professional runner listening to music? Have you ever wondered why that is?

It is a known fact that listening music during a run makes you lose focus. For an elite runner that seeks better results, it is necessary for him to be completely focused in order to monitor his body, since it must function like a precise machine. Any distractions might cause his pace to change or oscillate, which will cost him seconds at the end of the race. Are you planning to run in the Olympics? If so, then forgive me, because I'm not, and I want to keep listening to music during my workouts. I have run many times without listening to music, for a variety of reasons – running with a partner, having forgotten my equipment or simply no batteries. I *can* run without listening to music, but I do not like doing that.

As I previously mentioned when I was on the subject of gym wear, the same goes for electronics. You should be fine if you are using them for a walk, but if you are going to use them for long runs, you will have problems.

As any beginner runner does, I used that case with hook-and-loop fasteners in which you put your mobile phone and fasten it to your arm. That case is made of some kind of neoprene with a plastic cover for you to see and use your mobile phone. What they do not mention is that that case is not waterproof. In years of running, I have never found a 100% waterproof case.

The biggest enemy of sports equipment is sweat, and sadly our bodies sweat *a lot!* By the end of a long race, my running shoes and clothes are so drenched in sweat that I could wring them. Even that mobile phone case gets drenched in sweat.

When I started running, I realised that my mobile phone's sound system was failing. I noticed small signs of corrosion and rust in my earphones' plugs. I cleaned my phone's plug and bought new earphones. I kept using my phone and the problem persisted. I noticed that the volume buttons also started to fail, so I took it to technical support and for my surprise, the inside of my phone was covered in sweat. I looked everywhere for a waterproof phone case or for a way to make my phone waterproof. There exists no such thing, so I had to forget about using a mobile phone to run.

I could not use my phone, and consequently I could not monitor my runs and would not able to listen to music. Therefore, I started using a stopwatch and bought a cheap MP3 player just to listen to music. It was very interesting to learn how to use a stopwatch and how to calculate my runs. I learned a lot about pace, average speed and measurement conversion. In contrast, I had a terrible experience with second-hand MP3 players and allegedly waterproof earphones, which usually do not last more than a few runs, with batteries lasting only around forty minutes due to sweating. I had to run with my phone in my hands many times, which was not pleasant. I tried wearing a belt pack with my mobile phone inside it, but the result was chafing due to its straps and my phone was still drenched by the end of the run.

After some time, I noticed that one of the pleasures of running is the feeling of freedom and lightness, so carrying a mobile phone was starting to keep me from that feeling. I started trying not to carry too many things, so whenever I go to a race by car, I even hide my keys so that I do not have to carry them. It puzzles me when I see people carrying things such as squeezes and towels. The truth is that the less things you carry, the greater the feeling of freedom will be.

Sunglasses were also a disappointment to me, although I found it pleasant to walk whilst wearing them. When I started running farther, I realised that I would have to discard them, because in addition to being stained with sweat, it got blurry quickly. Whenever I decided to take sunglasses, I would have to carry them on my hands and that became a bore.

Unfortunately, all my equipment problems were solved by spending money. After a few months of running races, I bought a GPS watch, a Garmin Forerunner 220. I bought a used watch online, but what disappoints me is how much one has to pay for such an equipment. A similar or better watch would cost half the price in the United States, or even less. These products are too costly in Brazil.

A GPS watch will provide you with all information that any running app has, with the added benefit of not having to carry a mobile phone. I do not know nor can I say what is the best or worst watch that you can use to monitor your runs. I would say that the best one is the one that you can afford.

I solved my problem of lack of music by buying an iPod Shuffle and a zip lock bag. I chose that iPod due to the fact that its batteries lasts for more than five hours, which would allow me to run a marathon, and also because it is small enough to fit my pockets. I always put it inside the bag and close it, so that only its cord is out of the bag and it does not get wet.

I like wearing thick socks when running, especially when the weather is cold. These socks offer mid compression, which is good for the calf, and they also heat up the skin when it is cold and offer some degree of protection. When I ran on highways, I noticed that cars would launch pebbles on my legs, which could hurt me. The socks reduce these wounds, but it impossible to wear them on hot days. Ever since I started working out I got used to wearing thermal shorts, which are made of Lycra and replace underwear. I would wear them because as a result of being overweight, my inner thighs rubbed on each other during my walks, and thus I had skin chafing.

After a year of running, my equipment was composed of running shoes, thick socks, shorts, thermal shorts, dry fit t-shirts, hats, my Garmin watch and my iPod. On cold days, I would wear a compression long-sleeve shirt under my t-shirt and gloves. As my fingertips usually feel cold, I bought specific running gloves.

Your necessity to carry accessories or not will depend on the type of exercise that you do. If I am doing my daily workout, I usually do not bring anything besides my watch and my iPod. I do not even bring water, since my route begins and ends on my house. For up to a two-hour workout, I do not drink any water (please note that this is *my* habit, so you do not need to do the same).

I start having problems, though, when I went for long runs, which usually last three hours and a half. We do not have the option to run in parks with drinking fountains around running tracks in my area, so my long runs are done in the roadside of the Rio-Santos highway, either north or south. There are also no shops on the roadside, because most of them are still closed when I am working out. In such cases, I must take my belt pack with a water bottle to drink during my long runs. I also take an ID, my mobile phone and money in case something happens, but I store all of it in a tightly closed zip lock bag.

I mentioned this once, but I will repeat it: when going out for a long run in a more deserted place, it is extremely important to let someone know about your route, when you are leaving and when you are coming back, and take your phone or some means of communication. You must remember that unexpected things happen. You could injure yourself during a race when you are twenty kilometres away in a small road, in the middle of nowhere. Imagine not being able to walk and being isolated. If you have your mobile phone, you can even call a taxi or a private car to take you home.

It would be ideal if we could run without clothes on and without any accessories. A sweaty t-shirt is heavier and sticky, but without it you might get skin chafing and even sunburns. Running shoes are heavy, tight and hot, but without them your feet would have no extra soles and the lack of cushioning would destroy your joints. Shorts and tops are also heavy, tight and get drenched in sweat, but provide support and protect from chafing. Therefore, it is necessary to run fully-clothed. You should choose good-quality clothes and good accessories – they might cost more, but they are surely better than second-hand items.

MY FIRST MARATHON

The thrill of having completed my first half-marathon was so good that I wanted to experience it again. I registered for the 10th edition of the São Paulo International Half-Marathon, which was scheduled for February 2016. I hadaboutthreemonths to prepare for it.

This race would start and end on Charles Müller Square[12]. The route would pass by Elevado Costa e Silva (Minhocão)[13], República Square, Consolação Street, Av. Ipiranga, São JoãoAvenue,PacaembúAvenue, and soon. The race, organised by Yes.com, is supposed to be an invitation to visit São Paulo, since many touristic attractions and important landmarks are part of the route. It would certainly be one that I would like to participatein multiple times.

---

[13]Elevado Costa e Silva is a 3.50-kilometre elevated highway which connects the west area of Sao Paulo to the downtown and the south area. Its name was changed in 2016 after a law was passed changing names of all streets honouring people involved in the Brazilian Military Dictatorship (1964-1985). It is mostly known as "Minhocão" nowadays, an enormous earth-worm like creature.

I managed to prepare for the race without any surprises this time, so I finished the race on a better time than my first half-marathon, even though this one had slopes and downslopes, which alters the pace a lot. It wasindeed a greatrace.

Even before running this second half-marathon, I had registered for another one, the International Half-Marathon of São Paulo City, which was on its 17th edition and is organised by Corpore. Yes, there are two half-marathons with very similar names, but yet they are completely different races. This one would start and end inside the University of Sao Paulo (USP)[14], which is very close to my parents' house.

This race occurred in April 2016, so I only had an interval of two months between the races. I was very well prepared, but no one was expecting that the sun would shine so brightly on that morning. The air was very dry as it had not rained for weeks, and even though we were in April[15], it still seemed like we were in summer. In fact, the heat was so intense that I thought about giving up many times during that

---

[14] The University of São Paulo has its main campus in Butantã, which is known as "Cidade Universitária" ("University City") due to its sheer size of more than 7.44 square km². It has eleven campuses in the state of São Paulo, with four of them located in its capital city.

[15] The seasons in Brazil are the opposite from the Northern Hemisphere. Also, São Paulo in particular is known for its very unstable weather, no matter the season.

race. I recall having drunk a lot of water during the race, which was unusual, as well as washing my hair and face.

We ran on a part of Polytechnic Avenue, and because of the race, it was completely blocked off the rest of the campus. I believe that was not necessary, since all athletes ran on the sidewalk and under the shade of the wall surrounding USP due to the immense heat. It was 8 AM, but it seemed like it was 11 AM, since the asphalt was hot and no wind blew. This was the toughest race I ever ran, even though the distance was shorter than a marathon. After the race ended, most people said that it was so hot that it seemed like there was one shining sun for every participant – indeed, many athletes threw themselves on the grass surrounding the road in their exhaustion and I saw many people feeling sick. Perhaps the start should have been rescheduled to an hour earlier – still, who could have known *how* hot it would get?

After running these two half-marathons, I concluded that it was time to aim higher! I wanted more... I wanted to run a marathon... *I wanted to try the 42K race*!

I ranmost of myraces in São Paulo due to the simplefactthatmyparentslivethere and alsobecauseraces are heldalmostevery weekend. It was very practical for me to run in

São Paulo for a number of reasons: not only did I already know the city – which made it much easier to understand the routes and to get to the starting points – but I also had my family close by and I would have no expenses besides the trip. In fact, running in another city requires planning for transportation, hotels, places to eat, things to pack, etc. Therefore, I decided to run my first marathon in Sao Paulo. Unfortunately, I had heard only bad things about the São Paulo International Marathon: that it has a very dull route without passing by any historical places besides Ibirapuera Park, but I had no other option. It was most disappointing to know that that year's marathon had been held, so the next one would only be held a year later, on May 2017.

The fact that I would have to travel to be able to run a marathon in 2016 made me upset, since I could not have extra expenses at the time. However, I had a great surprise when I was looking up upcoming races. Asics and Iguana Sports were organising the first edition of Sao Paulo City Marathon, which would take place on July 31, 2016. I promptlyregistered for it and paid the fee. That was it, I was feeling butterflies in my stomach. *Let the 42K come!*

I had a good workout pace and was used to doing my spreadsheets and planning diets. I was able to control my weight and my pace was getting better and better. When I wastraining for my second half-marathon, I completed a long run of 33 kilometres from my house to Itamambuca beach, to the Caisão and back home. Finally, during my training for my third half-marathon, I completed another long run of 32 kilometres, from home to the Rio Escuro hill and back, through the highway. It did not seem hard to add ten kilometres to my runs. I had to focus and dedicate myself to my running goals, so I would create a new workout plan.

I had three months to train for the Marathon. In order to do so, I registered for two short races in the meantime: "Soldado Paulino", which was my first run – it is still one my favourite races – and Athenas 16K, which would take place two weeks before the marathon. It would be interesting for me to run Athenas 16K, since it would be a longer route just before the Marathon. As for "Soldado Paulino", though, I wanted to run it just for fun. Since it was only 10K, it would not interfere in my training, on the contrary, that race was a fartlek in my workout plan.

I kept my workouts organised. I did not skip any workouts; of course I reduced a few kilometres or changed my workout days, but I kept my schedule intact. I was also controlling my diet, so that my consumption of proteins, fibres and carbohydrates was balanced. I would weigh myself before and after working out.I would control my hydration levels and my workouts. I started doing abs almost daily and put my long-forgotten dumbbells to good use. My physical fitness and running posture improved a lot as a result of those abs exercises.

I was feeling prepared to do a long run before the race, which was that dumb idea of running farther before the race. Unfortunately, I would not have much time for that, soI would have to do it a few weeks before the race. This time, I wouldtry to cover 45K.

Therefore, I started setting routes on Google Maps and discovered that it would be possible to run to the nearby city of Caraguatatuba, more specifically to the Capricórnio beach.

I did a longrunsouthaftermyfirsthalf-marathon and reached the summit of Rio Escuro Hill, whichborders Dura beach. I ranthirty-twokilometres. It wasinterestingbecauseinitially I hadjustwanted to try a new routewith no expectations, since I didnottakeanywater, moneynormyphone.

I remembered that a friend of mine, Pedrinho, told me that when he used to run, he would go as far as Saco da Ribeira once every two months. I thoughtthatwasimpressive, so I wanted to try it myself. I aimedmyrunningshoes to the Southern beaches and startedrunning. I passedbyPraia Grande, Toninhas, Enseada, Perequê-mirim and finallyreachedSaco da Ribeirabeach. I pressedon to Lázaro until I wasdefeatedby the slope of Rio Escuro Hill, which is high. What I like the most about it is that there is a fountain a few metres before the descent. I drankwater and returned home.

The fact that I had already done this workout gave me the idea of going all the way to the Military Police station in Tabatinga beach in Caraguatatuba. Unfortunately, it would not be enough – only thirty-four kilometres, which was eight kilometres less than the distance of the race and also eleven kilometres less than my goal. I decided to stick to the idea of passing by the police station and to continue on to the Capricórnio beach, which would add a good amount of slope – the hill between Caraguatatuba and Ubatuba.

I intended to do it like usual: leave my house at dawn and by the time the sun rosethere would be less than a third of the route to cover. I would take a 700ml squeeze with Gatorade, money, my ID, my mobile phone, my iPod and my

Garmin. Wheneverythingwasready, I started feeling excited. This time, I would cover a much longer distance than the longest of my runs.

I woke up at four in the morning on that day. I got dresses and put food for Vicky and for my cat. I left and stretched three times. At this moment the penny dropped and I realised what I was about to do. I turned the sound on and started running.

During a longrun, onehas time to think of manythings. One has enough time to think about many problems, remember things, plan routines and attitudes. In my opinion, it is very important to control your thoughts during a long run, since you will need a lot of psychological strength to endure running for hours. Since I am not an elite nor a professional athlete, running is a pleasure to me and I do not believe in that saying about focusing on the run. I prefer distracting my thoughts to focus on other things, so it does not become boring. I am always monitoring my pace and distance using my Garmin watch and that is enough for me – I do not need to focus on my breath, heartbeats and so on. I would rather think about my life and its events. I like to use that running time to think about my problems. I let my body go on its own way, perhaps even better than if I were worried about breathing correctly and keeping my pace at each step. That is how I was able to run many kilometres.

The route chosen had many slopes and one of them was indeed difficult: the Rio Escuro Hill slope. I had climbed it once, and on that day, when I finished it, I decided that I would try it again, for I was feeling exhausted at the time. On my second try, not only would I have to climb it, but I would also have to run twenty-five kilometres afterwards. The first slope of the route was short, but steep – the Praia Grande lookout slope. The second was longer and steeper, it was the hill that divided Toninhas and Enseada beaches. Before reaching Saco da Ribeira beach, there was also a mound with turns and slopes. After that we have the feared Rio Escuro Hill. The last slope would be after the Military Police base in Tabatinga beach.

I covered the first stretch of the route until the end of Toninhas beach on a slower pace as a warm-up exercise. I wasn't tired when I faced the hill to Enseada beach. As soon as I finished my descent and arrived in Enseada, I felt good and I felt confident, since this was the second highest hill of the route. There were only unending straight stretches of road until Saco da Ribeira, which meant that I had to avoid eventual bikers and pedestrians on the roadside. After running in the turns and mounds that make way for Saco da Ribeira, I felt a bit tired and finally took a sip of my Gatorade.

My biggest challenge was starting to show itself on the end of the straight road I was running on. A smooth left curve and a ramp appeared before my eyes. The road continued upwards until it did an "S" shape and disappeared behind a curve. I stomped my foot soles on the asphalt, took shorter steps, inclined my body and started a new pace for that slope that was longer than a kilometre. I ran each metre, curve by curve of that road that seemed to only end in the sky. After agonising breaths, I finally reached the summit and the fountain. I stopped for a moment to wash my mouth, since it was dry and salty. Now I had to descend the slope. I had never run farther than that slope, so it was a new experience to me. To my astonishment, I found that going down the hill was not so steep, but it was a very long way. I covered a few kilometres in my descent, which gave me time to recompose myself.

I had run more than twenty kilometres and was running on the unending straight road of Lagoinha beach, and then another one in Maranduba beach. At that point, the sun was shining and the heat of the asphalt was starting to bother me. I haddrunkwater a few times.

When I reached the 32K mark and reached the edge of town, which is on the border between the two cities, I felt completely exhausted. All of a sudden, my legs weakened and I walked sluggishly. I felt like my legs weighed tonnes. I drank what liquid was left on my squeeze and tried to focus on the run and pressed on, step by step.

At thirty-three kilometres, I had no more feet, only anvils were stuck to my shins. Each step I took was a sacrifice. Perhaps I could go faster if I switched to walking.

I reached the Military Police base at thirty-four kilometres. "I reached my goal", I thought. I walked five hundred metres and placed my hand on the *wall!* And now I couldn't take another step. I was too exhausted. I doubled over and put my hands on my knees. There was no pain. I was okay, but awfully exhausted, as if my last breath had been taken away from me.

I checked my Garmin: "Distance: 34.5 km". I had not managed to reach my goal. In that moment, I felt disappointed. I had failed. Many bad things crossed my mind then, but mostly that there would be no time for a new test. I would have to run forty-two kilometres in that race, with no preliminary tests. I wasscared.

After a few minutes standing still and breathing, I recomposed myself and started walking back, or perhaps dragging myself back to the Military Police base. I found a faucet in the station's garden and washed my face. I returned a few more metres in the highway and found the bus stop, where I'd take the bus back home.

I waited for that bus for more than an hour. I was tired, sweaty, hungry, thirsty and especially upset for not having been able to complete my goal, so what I wanted the most was to get home. I was tired of waiting, so I walked to the edge of town, since some buses also passed by there and one of them could take me home. I walked for twenty minutes to the next bus stop. This time, it did not take long for the bus to come.

I must admit that I was impressed with the distance I had run, even though I was sad for having failed, I felt proud, since it was an impressive feat. At least I didn'tknowanyonewhohadalreadydone it.

By the time I got home, I had realised that I had been very wrong in the organisation of my long run. I should have gone by bus and returned running. Had I done that, I would probably be home, fed, clean and probably asleep. I drank some water and took a shower. I changed, got something to eat and laid down on my couch. I started watching TV and feel asleep in a few minutes. I wastotallyexhausted.

I sticked to my workout plan and to my diet on the the following days. The Athenas 16K race took place two weeks after the long run. Aneasy, simplerace and a straightroute. Eight kilometres walking on Marginal Pinheiros to go and eight more kilometres to return. That's it. It was an excellent race, in which I did not feel tired nor did I feel any pain. I was ready for the marathon, which would take place in two weeks.

When I participated in the two shorter races that preceded the marathon, I was very fit, perhaps on my best shape. I weighedseventykilos. I coveredbothrouteson a lessthan 5 minutes pace. I hit a personal record for ten kilometres during Athenas 16K (which would be broken after the marathon in an unpretentious workout in my backyard). In the "Soldado Paulino" race, I reached the 17th place in my age group. I needn't say that these positive results made me more confident for the marathon. Still, one thing bothered me: *I had not completed my long run.*

The two weeks after Athenas 16K flew and it was finally the day to go to São Paulo. This time, I wentby car. On that Saturday, after work, I stopped by my house, got my bag and went to São Paulo. I arrived at my parents' house at around 9 PM, which would give me enough time to sleep. It was agreed that my mother would take me to the starting point at Charles Müller Square.

The São Paulo City Marathon had a routethatincluded a goodportion of the São Paulo International Half-Marathon. It also passed by the Minhocão and the Republic Square, but then towards Sé Square, São Francisco Plaza, Paulista Avenue, Jardins, Ibirapuera, the São Paulo Jockey Club, Panamericana Square, Villa-Lobos Park, USP and it would finally end on the Jockey Club. I should not forget to mention the feared slope in Brigadeiro Luís Antonio Avenue. Thiswassuch a huge tour throughSâo Paulo.

I woke up at four in the morning and quickly got dressed, since I had prepared everything the day before. I do not like preparing things at the last minute, so I always attach my bib number to the t-shirt that I will wear. I always charge my iPod and my watch, and set out my clothes as well as the documents to take. I usually take one of these bags that are gifted to us on the races, with everything I need inside it, such as my ID, keys, mobile phone, money, a small towel. After I was ready, I went to wake up my mother, but to my surprise she was almost ready. We left an hour and a half before the race. This time, I knew that I wouldn't be able to get very close to the starting point.

We drove throughRebouças Avenue and took the tunnel to access Pacaembú. When we started going down the hill which gives access to Charles Müller Square, we found ourselves stuck in traffic, since Pacaembú Avenue was already blocked. I asked my mother to return and drop me off there. We agreed that I would call her after finishing the race, so that she could pick me up at Jockey Club. I walked in the direction of the starting point, mingling with the hundreds of runners that appeared on the surrounding streets. When I reached the top of the stairs before the Square, I saw a colourful sea of runners getting ready for the race. It was still dark and spotlights illuminated the crowd.

In the starting point was the usual, but in greatquantity. There were hundreds of stalls with sports equipment, as well as sports consultancy stalls. Hundreds of public toilets, and many buses that were like lockers, since they would eventually go to the Jockey Club with participants' belongings and part of the staff. Although the environment was contagious, I was really apprehensive. I stored my belongings on a bus and tried to locate my starting point. I started stretching, which this time was done more carefully and repeated a few times.

The São Paulo City Marathon was started as "Satisfaction" by Rolling Stones played. I had planned to keep a 5'40" pace for at least thirty-five kilometres, and I would start drinking water at the twenty-five kilometre mark. I had four maltodextrin energy gels to consume at twenty, twenty-seven, thirty, thirty-five and forty kilometres. I wanted to feel the environment of the race, so I decided to run with iPod turned off for half the race, that is, until Jockey Club.

The crowd carries us during the first few kilometres, but it is vital to avoid fooling yourself with the paces of surrounding athletes. It is crucial to pay attention to one's pace during these first kilometres. Thatwilltake its tolllater in the race.

I ran happily, observing everything and excited about the environment of the race. The view of São Paulo at night is very interesting and running though those century-old streets was a privilege. When we ran through the most famous corner of São Paulo, Ipiranga Avenue and São João Avenue, we came across a present that the event staff prepared for us. The singing group TrovadoresUrbanos was serenading us, singing "Sampa[16]" for the athletes. It was fantastic.

This present was repeated a few more times throughout the route. There was an orchestra at the Municipal Theatre and a DJ down the hill at Brigadeiro Luis Antonio. In Ibirapuera Park we saw an Italian dance group performing Tarantellas, and a Japanese group playing the drums. Wesaw a chorinho[17]group in Villa-Lobos Park and a percussiongroupusingcansat USP.I believe that the staff did very well to place those attractions along the route. It was very encouraging for me.

I ran through the Old Town with no added difficulty. After running around São Paulo Plaza and passing by the Law School of the University of São Paulo, it was time to face the slope of Brigadeiro Luis Antonio Avenue, which ends on Paulista Avenue. I must admit that when I faced that ramp, I thought nothing of it, since the slope of the Rio Escuro Hill was much worse. I climbed that slope with no difficulty. I crossed

---

[16] One of the most famous, popular songs honouring São Paulo. It was composed by leading Brazilian singer Caetano Veloso in 1978. "Sampa" is also an affectionate nickname for the city.

[17] Chorinho ("little cry" or "little lament") is an instrumental Brazilian popular music genre which originated in Rio de Janeiro during the 19th century. Despite its name, the music usually consists of happy, fast rhythm.

Paulista Avenue and now it was time to go down to Ibirapuera Park. After a climb, there is always a way down.

In thatmoment, I noticedthat a man in histhirtiesstartedaccompanyingmypace. This is very common in road races; an athlete runs beside another and it is common for groups of athletes to run together, which we call running teams.

I did not mind, since having a distraction or someone struggling with me would give me added strength in my steps. I never knew the name of that runner, since we barely greeted each other.

The first "distance split" took place at Ibirapuera Park. Those that wished to complete the marathon would need to continue on until they ran around the Obelisk, and those that were running half of it would return. I quickly realised that only a few completed the marathon. I could count on my fingertips the number of athletes that I found in that stretch of the route. After running around the Obelisk, I mingled again with the crowd and entered Juscelino Kubitschek Avenue, in the direction of the tunnel.

The aforementioned tunnel connects Juscelino Kubitschek Avenue to near the entrance of the Jockey Club. It was the end of the race for those that were running the half-marathon, but for some of us, it was awful. It was indeed the most difficult part of the race. It started as a steep slope down to a very long climb up, which became quite steep in the end. I knew that this was a very steep climb due to ache in my legs. I had never noticed that whilst driving through that tunnel and there was no data about this tunnel on the marathon website. It wasindeedcomplicated.

When I left the tunnel and startedrunningthrough the avenuewhere the Jockey Club is located, near USP, I felt a bit jealous of thosethatwerereturning to enter its arena and finish the race. I still had twenty-one kilometres to go, the same distance I had already covered.

I kept on with my unnamed partner through that avenue, then across Cidade Universitária Bridge, Panamericana Square, Pedroso de Moraes Avenue and Villa-Lobos Park. When we reached the entrance to the park, my partner complained that he'd stop, since he couldn't take it anymore. I toldhim to lowerourpacesothathecouldfinish the race. My pace, which was 5'45" at the time, fell to 5'55". I was thankful because I could blame him for having lowered our pace and not the fact that I was also tired.

My legs started to hurt when I was about to enter USP, having run more than thirty-two kilometres. I had already drank water and used my energy gels, and still I felt that I was out of breath. As soon as we entered the campus' main avenue, my partner broke down.

He was almost crying and out of breath when he told me to keep going, as he needed to stop. Judging by his expressions and grunts during the last few kilometres, he was indeed struggling and had given it his all. I said goodbye, promising to meet him at the finish line, which never happened.

Now that I was running alone again, I turned up my iPod's volume, which I had only turned on when I was in front of the Jockey Club. I tried to get back to my previous pace, but it was impossible. After running for thirty-five kilometres, my pace was 6 minutes per kilometre. I was now running through the unending forested streets of USP. It is very annoying to run at USP, because the landscape never changes, all you can see are trees and straight streets for kilometres. There is nothingelse to see. I believethat I had no more patienceatthat point.

I reached the thirty-seven kilometre mark with much effort. I suddenlyfelt a tremor onmy posterior legmuscles, akin to involuntaryspasm. I hadneverfeltanythinglikethat. I pressedon for a few more hundred metres and then I felt it.I felt that incandescent knitting needle in my thigh again – this time, four times in a row, like four bee stings at the same time. I felt a very strong spasm on my leg and it contracted in a mixture of pain and muscle cramps. I did not hit the *wall* this time, it fell over me. I doubled over and touched my thigh. I pressed it and it hurt.

The São Paulo City Marathon was over for me.

I wanted to cry because I was in pain and tired, but mostly I wanted to cry in frustration. I could not admit that it was over. I tried to run again, but the pain hit me again as soon as I set my feet on the ground. It was less intense, but it was still enough for me to understand that the race was over for me.

I had to resort to walking the rest of the route. A motorbike with medical attention stopped by and asked me if I was fine, I said yes and that I was only resting. They left. I kept walking until I got to the next hydration stop, a few hundred metres ahead of where I had broken down.

I drank a bottle of Gatorade and took one for later. Seeing that big ice barrel gave me an idea. I took a big ice block and put in on my thigh, and I walked as I pressed the ice on my thigh and drank more Gatorade. After a few minutes, my leg felt better and the pain diminished. I tried to jog for a bit and realised that the pain was tolerable.

I took ice blocks at every stop and put them on my thigh, whose skin was numb by then. My hand was also numb, but that did not matter, as I wanted to cross that finish line and would do that no matter what.

I ran the remaining kilometres inside USP and entered the last lane of the race. There were just a few kilometres left on the Jockey avenue and that was it.

When I left that avenue and entered the narrow street that gave access to the Arena, I felt another spasm in my calf, which meant another muscle cramps. My body showed many signs of exhaustion. When I saw the finish line only a few metres away, emotion overcame me. A mixture of struggle, pain, pride and achievement took over me and I tried to raise my arms as in a celebration gesture, but I could not – the muscles on my legs and back reacted, so that I could not raise my arms higher than my head. I was completely exhausted, but I had completed the race.

I crossed the finish line after four hour and forty minutes of running and struggling. My final pace was 6'06".

When the promoter put the medal around my neck, it seemed to weight one tonne, for my body leaned forward. I had to find somewhere to rest. I followed the crowd to the lockers, I recovered my bag and I rested on the Jockey Club's bleachers. I sat there for more than an hour, with a blank look, just breathing. I fearedthat I wouldnotbeable to stand up. After resting, I called my mother and asked her to pick me up outside the Jockey Club.

During that hour of resting, sitting on the bleachers of the Jockey Club – it was a nice place to be after finishing a marathon, since on those lanes before me ran the real running machines of nature: horses – I thought over the race I had just completed.

I now had that wonderful post-marathon sensation that only those who run marathons will know and understand. It is anundescribable feeling of fulfilment and happiness. I thoughtabout the lastyear and a half of mylife. I recalled seeing that man, as light as a shade, almost floating as he ran on the shore of Itaguá beach, telling those women to run if they really wanted to lose weight, until the last metres of the marathon.

It had been a year and a half of dedication, discipline and mostly, of change. I realised howrunningbrought me muchneededphysical and mental health. How many times had I given up eating delicious foods to achieve that which I had *just* achieved? That medal on my chest meant so much more than running forty-two kilometres. It mean a new lease of life ahead that had begun to change a year and a half before. Every drop of sweat, every lettuce leaf eaten, every toenail that fell and every woken moment at dawn to train were thusly assembled, represented and crowned by that medal, by that achievement. I was very happy mostly because I had not given up on myself in one of the hardest moments of my life. As I sat alone at the Jockey Club bleachers, with a huge medal pending from my neck, I started crying.

CONCLUSION

In these years since I started losing weight and dedicating myself to running, I ran thousands of kilometres in workouts and races. I participated in many road races. I improved my running technique and started spending money in better running equipment. I practicallychangedmylifestyle. I become a marathoner.

I can guarantee one thing: anyone healthy that dedicate themselves are able to complete a marathon, and it is such a unique sensation to cross that finish line. When I registered for my first marathon, I did not imagine that it would be such a "gorilla". I waswrong, though. A marathon is not a "gorila", it is a King Kong.

I willsay the following, without a doubt: completingmyfirstmarathonwas the biggesteffort I made in mylifeuntilnow. I cannotrememberanysituation in which I triedharderorstruggledsomuch. For thatreason, I herebydiscourageadventurers, as marathoning is not for everyone. Onlythosewho are qualified are able to finish it. It is not possible to finish a marathon without adequate training nor without good mental and physical preparation.It is even dangerous to go on that odyssey without adequate preparation.

Many interesting things crossed my mind while I was sitting on those bleachers after finishing my first marathon. I watched a film of myliferegardingmylastyear and a half, in which I changedmanyaspects of myroutine. I feltenvelopedbygoodenergies. All of it was fantastic, but there was something that would not leave my mind and kept bugging me until I returned to Ubatuba. *I didnotfinish the race!*

It was beautiful to place my medal in my restaurant for my customers to admire, but the fact that I had broken down was always on my mind. I walked. I cheated. My sole rule for races was very simple: I had to cover the distance without walking. I had only walked for one kilometre during the marathon, but that still counted as walking, so I was out of the fame. In my opinion, I had not managed to complete the race, no matter what anyone said. I nowhadone more reason to do mybest in myworkouts. My new goal was to cover the distance of that marathon without walking – not even a metre. Even though people would say what I did was enough and that it didn't have to be like that, I was not convinced. It *had* to be the way I wanted! That is justhowlife is.

The fact that I took the initiative to start to lose weight, and afterwards walking, running, participating in road races and then participating in a marathon was due to something simple, which moves everything in the world: willpower. All the changes and subsequente achievements in my life were consequences of my willpower. It is not enough to have an idea as it is necessary to execute it, to put it in practice. In order to achieveallyouwant in life, you must dedicateyourself to it. One must notletlazinessdefeatthem; one must lowertheirhead in humility and make it happen. This is not to say that you are never going to wish to give up – that will eventually happen, but it is like my friend Zildo Lopes once said: "run to that sign, then to that pole. Whenyourealise it, it willbe over. Yourtiredness is gone". He is right. One cannot give up nor fool themselves with the thoughts that make them stop. In order to achieve more, one must never be satisfied with what they already have.

After I started running, I found that I needed to change many things, such as bad habits or wrong customs that held me back in life. I had to persist to overcome many of them, for laziness always hindered me. Although I overcame most of my difficulties, I am still struggling with many of them.

Nowadays, I keep working out to run marathons. I now have the goal of participating in international marathons. Who knows? I maybeable to complete the SixMajors. A dream, yousay? Perhaps, but I believe that we can achieve anything as long as we have willpower. For instance, I, in this moment, am facing one of my toughest battles yet: I am trying to stop smoking… Oh yes, I had forgotten to mention that throughout this book. I smokecigarettes. I smoke one pack of cigarettes a day, but I am trying to stop and I am sure that I will be able to do it. *Focus!*

TIPS

I will try to introduce here a series of tips that can and will help you a lot when you are trying to overcome, let's say, the "feeding abstinence" and the laziness. These are verysimplethingsthatcangivewill more quality of life. Although many of these tips might seem too simple, funny, a bit absurd, they work. It is worth a try.

SET A CERTAIN WEIGHT AS YOUR GOAL. It is important to have a goal to reach. This number should be remain carved in your mind so that you will never feel satisfied after losing a few kilos. "I lostfivekilos. Okay, that is good... but I still have twenty kilos to go." This is howyouwillfocus.

HAVE A SCALE IN YOUR TOILET OR BATHROOM. Also, weigh yourself everyday when you wake up and before going to bed. Do it without any clothes on. I also weigh myself before and after working out.

SLEEP EARLY. I have always believed that it is best to exercise early in the morning, as soon as I wake up. However, in order to wake up early, it is vital that you sleep early. An added benefit of sleeping early is that we do not eat while we sleep. The longer we stay awake, the more the body will need sustenance and the more food it will demand. Try to sleepatleasteight hours a day.

TRY TO EXERCISE IN THE MORNING. I like running with sunrise, so that is why I tend to get up around five in the morning. Furthermore, running, especially long runs, demands time to train. I leave to run at five thirty in the morning and finish around seven o'clock. Finally, another fact that makes me believe that the best time to run is as soon as I get up is that my mind is empty of the problems that we gather throughout the day. When I close my business for the day, I like going home to rest, without any more obligations or tasks. If I end up running at the end of the day, I do not perform as well as I could, because I will have felt annoyed, upset about something or worried. I am still not mentally tired when I wake up, so that is why I prefer running on that part of the day: I can be more focused on my exercise.

DRINK A LOT OF WATER. We know how important it is to keep one's body hydrated, but another secret is that drinking a large glass of water many times a day reduces hunger. A glass of sugar-free soft drink can fool your stomach for a while. I am not saying that you should only drink water or drink a sugar-free soft drink and exercise right away, but drinking a large glass of a sugar-free beverage when you are desperately wanting to devour a chocolate box can indeed put out a fire.

OCCUPY YOUR FREE TIME. Returning to an old hobby might be a way of keeping your mind busy in a moment of leisure, when you would probably turn to that BIS[18] box inside your cupboard. Any hobby, especially manual hobbies, distracts the mind from hunger and it keeps your hands busy. This could be excellent help for concentration, as well as a fantastic pastime. When our minds and hands are occupied, we tend to forget the will to eat.

AVOID GOING TO PLACES WHERE YOU WILL WANT TO EAT. Why suffer? It is hard enough to not be able to eat your favourite foods, so why visit the shopping centre's food court?

ALWAYS LEAVE HOME ON A FULL STOMACH. This is a good tip for when we go to a dinner party or to a birthday party, where we know that we will have to eat something that isn't part of the diet. Well, my technique for not exaggerating is to leave home after having eaten a meal. You will eat, moderately. Even when one is in a diet it is difficult to eat with no hunger, as delicious as the food may be.

---

[18] Popular Brazilian chocolate brand. It belongs to LAKA.

DO NOT GO SHOPPING WHEN YOU'RE HUNGRY. This tip will help you save money. Never go to the supermarket when you are hungry, since you will put things in your cart that you don't need. It is much more rational to go shopping to replenish food, without being hungry. That way you won't bring home that light biscuit nor that condensed milk can which you have not seen for weeks.

LOOK AT YOURSELF IN THE MIRROR. You should have mirrors spread around your home. Put a mirror in your bedroom, so that you can see your body as soon as you get up. Put a mirror in your toilet so that you will see yourself without clothes every day. You should love your body – admire it and criticise it. Embarrass yourself of the way it looks now and strengthen your will to change that. You should be able to see the body that you long for.

DO NOT HAVE FOOD AT HOME. Perhaps this is the greatest tip of all... when we are dieting, we all become MacGyvers in the kitchen. I love eating and cooking. For me, finding a lost can of condensed milk and a packet of Cream Cracker biscuits meant that I would bake a dessert. I am saying this for you to see how dangerous it is to have any "forgotten" food at home. You should have nothing but the necessary ingredients for your diet. Put small quantities of fruit in your fridge, since it is not worth it to have apples in the fridge and eat twelve of them at once. Therefore, you should have little food and rations of it. The best way of avoiding eating unhealthy food is *to not have it at home.*

DO NOT IDLE ON THE STREET. When you leave home, you should leave to do an activity, such as working, studying, going to the gym, visiting friends. Our homes are our safe haven, our headquarters. This is why taking a stroll on the street will make you hungry sooner or later and there are various temptations and many options to choose from. If you get hungry, go back home, where you will have all the things that you can eat.It is best to be safe than sorry.

DO NOT BE DISCOURAGED IF YOU MAKE A MISTAKE. If one day you give in to the temptation and eat what you shouldn't, do not worry. Stick to your diet on the next day and focus, but not as if nothing happened. It is important that you feel guilty. The more you blame yourself, the less likely you will be to make a mistake again.

EAT FRUIT AND SALAD. There are no kinds of food with less calories than vegetables and fruit, so you can eat as much as you want. You should always have a piece of fruit in your fridge for a late night snack.

TAKE VITAMINS. It is always good to complete your diet with daily vitamin supplement pills.

SAVE A FEW CALORIES FOR LATE NIGHT SNACKS. If you are on a 1,000-calorie diet, save two hundred calories for a last meal before bed. It is awful to go to bed hungry and most times hunger even keeps us from sleeping. That is why it is important to have some calories saved so that you can grab a bite to eat a few minutes before going to bed. In addition, I also usually drink a glass of a sugar-free drink, which makes me feel more satiated.

HAVE SIMPLE SNACKS IN THE FRIDGE. I still tend to open my fridge to get something to eat, so in order to solve this problem without messing up your diet, you should have simple snacks on the fridge, such as fruit. You can have unpeeled, cut up pineapple in your fridge, so you can eat a slice every time you open the fridge. For instance, you can chop up carrots with olive oil and salt, or perhaps you can eat sweet grapes. You can keep eating late night snacks, but with healthy food.

PAY ATTENTION TO WHAT YOU EAT BEFORE WORKING YOU. It is quite common not to think about your dinner on the night before working out. When I do that, I usually have cramps when exercising. If you get to know your body, you will know what kinds of food are good for you when you run.

IF YOU ARE NOT FEELING WELL, DON'T RUN. If you are not feeling well, or if you are feeling some kind of discomfort, avoid running. Running takes its toll on the body, so pain can get worse on a run. Abdominal paincanbecomediarrhea. It is best to take the day off and train more when you are feeling better. You do not need to push yourself so hard, so running should make you feel good.

ONLY WEAR BRANDS THAT YOU LIKE. I usually stick to my favourite brands because I'm afraid that if I buy different and do not like it, I will never get my money back. When I buy something that I like, I avoid buying something else, such as my running shoes. I always buy the same, newer ones. If something isn't broken, do not fix it. I think this is a good tip for accessories, clothes, and even food and drink during races. Only use and wear what you like and are used to.

NEVER TRY RUNNING EQUIPMENT FOR THE FIRST TIME DURING A RACE. This is obvious. Never try running equipment for the first time during a race. If you want to wear new sneakers for a marathon, make sure that you have worn it during your workouts. New sneakers may cause blisters, a new t-shirt may cause allergies, and new shorts and tops may cause chafing. A new energy gel mightmakeyoufeelsick. Tryon new things in yourworkouts.

PROTECT YOUR EQUIPMENT FROM SWEAT. No mobile phone is 100% waterproof nor immune to the corrosive effects of sweat. I had serious problems due to carrying my phone around in one of those phone cases that you can find in any store. Although they might be useful for a walk, they are not useful for running for hours. I could not find any way to make my phone waterproof, so I had to change it for a GPS watch, and I started listening to music on an iPod Shuffle, which I could store inside a zip lock plastic bag.

CARRY AS FEW THINGS AS POSSIBLE. As running makes you feel free, the less things you carry during exercising, the best will that feeling be. I started discarding things for the fact that they were not useful anymore. My sunglasses got blurry, so I stopped wearing them. My mobile phone would get wet with my sweat, so I left it at home. I only brought a belt pack with a squeeze for long runs because I would drink water, but then I started drinking water at home, so

I stopped carrying it. I neverusedtowels. Therefore, I stopped carrying somanythings.

PLAN AHEAD BEFORE GOING ON LONG RUNS. When you leave for a long run, make sure to let someone know beforehand. Carry your mobile phone, ID, and money. You should always have a way to go back home, and always be ready for the unexpected. Avoid going on long runs in places that you have never been to or in notoriously dangerous places.

RESPECT YOUR BODY'S LIMITS. Training a lot does not equal exaggerating. You may find yourself paying a high price for excess training, so learn how to read your body's signs and understand its limits.

PLAN AHEAD FOR YOUR RACES. When you register for a race, start focusing on it. Take it seriously. Use that as a reason to train more and better. Letthatpre-raceanxietygrow and becomeexpectation. You should create workout spreadsheets and complete them accordingly. You should respect your dietary plan and the rules you set up. On the day of the race, set out your clothes and your things before leaving and prepare everything so that you will not be late.

TELL PEOPLE, DIVULGE YOUR DEEDS. Do not be embarrassed of telling your deeds to everyone. You will surely be praised and criticised, so you should take to heart what is good for you. Remember the comments that make you feel proud of yourself.

INVITE YOUR FRIENDS FOR A RUN. Tell people about your experience and encourage those of your friends that want to start running. Invite them for some light workout, so you will have a good time and you will also help someone. I always say that "Running is a solo sport." Even though I have running partners for workouts and even races. I can guarantee that I run alone 95% of the time. So it is really fun when a friend joins me, since I know that will not happen many times at all.

HAVE "YOUR" RUNNING GROUNDS. It is interesting to have a route that you always stick to, which will always be a reference when comparing times and distances. Find yourself a route which you are familiar with its every single metre. You will thusly feel comfortable to sprint and to test new workouts.

PAY ATTENTION TO YOUR PACE AT THE STARTING POINT OF A RACE. This is very important, since carelessness at the beginning of a race can take its toll by the end of it. In all races there are those who are really running and those who are in it just for fun. This second group are those that dash from the start and pass by you as quick as a rocket, or they stop for selfies, which disturbs and confuse the pace of those in the first group, the actual runners. In other words, always focus on your pace on the start of a race and do not let such people fool you. ATENTE-SE AO SEU RITMO NA LARGADA DE UMA PROVA.

APPRECIATE THE RACE. When you are running a race, appreciate the route, the environment of the race, and the landscape. Last but not least, use whatever services or attractions that event staff offers during the race.

ENJOY THE RACE. When we are running, there seems to be a moment when the body enters into an automatic mode. In that mode, breathing becomes regular, heartbeats became regular and so do each step. There is no pain. The brainseems to bewelloxygenated. In that moment, you become a passenger of your own body, since there is some kind of numbness in it. If you manage to clear your mind and your thoughts as soon as you feel that, you will enter a kind of trance, which causes a very good feeling.